Ethical Practi
in Brain Injury
Rehabilitation

Ethical Practice in Brain Injury Rehabilitation

Joanna Collicutt McGrath

Heythrop College
University of London

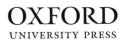

OXFORD
UNIVERSITY PRESS

OXFORD
UNIVERSITY PRESS

Great Clarendon Street, Oxford OX2 6DP

Oxford University Press is a department of the University of Oxford.
It furthers the University's objective of excellence in research, scholarship,
and education by publishing worldwide in

Oxford New York

Auckland Cape Town Dar es Salaam Hong Kong Karachi
Kuala Lumpur Madrid Melbourne Mexico City Nairobi
New Delhi Shanghai Taipei Toronto

With offices in

Argentina Austria Brazil Chile Czech Republic France Greece
Guatemala Hungary Italy Japan Poland Portugal Singapore
South Korea Switzerland Thailand Turkey Ukraine Vietnam

Oxford is a registered trade mark of Oxford University Press
in the UK and in certain other countries

Published in the United States
by Oxford University Press Inc., New York

A catalogue record for this title is available from the British Library
Data available

Library of Congress Cataloging in Publication Data
Data available

Typeset by Cepha Imaging Private Ltd., Bangalore, India
Printed in Great Britain
on acid-free paper by
Ashford Colour Press Ltd., Gosport, Hampshire

ISBN 978–0–19–856899–5 (Pbk.)

10 9 8 7 6 5 4 3 2 1

Contents

Acknowledgements

Over the years conversations with several colleagues have helped me in my thinking about ethical practice. In particular I would like to acknowledge Julie Elsworth, Patrick Haggard, Caroline Shackleton, and Ann Stead.

Tony Hope, Helen Liepman, Susan Oxbury, and Derick Wade gave me encouragement during the early stages of planning this book.

Conversations with Emlyn Hooson, Lesley Lambert, and Ashley Rogers pointed me in fruitful directions as it took shape.

Audrey Daisley, Catherine Epps, Nicola Proffit, and Rachel Tams took part in detailed and significant discussions on clinical and ethical issues that informed several of the case studies. I thank them for their professional wisdom, their willingness to share some of it with me, and for many times of laughter along the way.

I am grateful to Jan Quinlan for giving permission to reproduce two extracts of her work *An Abnormal Reality* - the second quote at the beginning of Chapter 2 and the longer cited extract later in that chapter.

It will be obvious from the text that I owe an overwhelming debt of gratitude to a large number of people with acquired brain injury, their families, friends, and carers, who have allowed me to interview them over a period of many years. This book is dedicated to them in recognition of their dignity, resilience, and courage.

Chapter 1

Introduction

Contemporary ethicists entertain theories about human nature, explore the nature of value, discuss competing accounts of the best way to live, ponder the connections between ethics and human psychology, and discuss practical ethical quandaries.

LaFollette (2000, p. 1)

1.1 An afternoon in the life of a neurological rehabilitation unit

It is Tuesday afternoon and I am seeing the last client of my outpatient clinic, Alison. Her husband, Brian, sustained a severe head injury in a fall 2 years ago. After a long period of rehabilitation he was discharged home to his family. He needs supervision for most activities of daily life, and he attends a day centre once a week. The couple are in their forties and have two children.

After a discussion of the results of her husband's neuropsychological assessment Alison tells me that she would like to ask some further questions concerning his psychology. She tells me that before the accident he was a loving husband and a very involved family man. He provided her with a good deal of emotional support. She describes him as a best friend as well as a lover. Both of them had strong religious beliefs and were involved in their local church. She continues,

> Since the accident he is so deeply changed. It's not just that he has difficulty walking and his memory is so bad. It's as if he has stopped loving us. All he thinks about is himself. He seems to have no emotions except anger if he can't have things immediately. It's like having another child in the house. He doesn't care about the children—he doesn't speak to them except to tell them to shut up. They don't say much but I notice they spend more time in their rooms and they don't invite friends home any more. He won't make love to me. The other day I told him I was upset about it and he just asked if I wanted to divorce him—he didn't seem that bothered about it. I'm so lonely [she starts to cry]. When he woke up from the coma we were so full of hope, but at times now I wish he'd never woken up—that's wrong, isn't it?' [I say nothing in

response but encourage her to continue telling me about her situation. This is probably good practice, but actually I can't think of anything to say.] I could cope with all
his physical problems, if there was just some sign of warmth or affection from him.

There's an old friend of mine, a widower we both know from our church. He has
been like a rock to me these past months. I don't know how I would have coped without him. I'm starting to develop feelings for him. But that must be wrong too mustn't
it? [Again I treat the question as rhetorical]

I've been wondering about what my marriage means. I believe in the sanctity of
marriage. When you make those vows you promise to stay with your husband for better
for worse, in sickness and in health. But what if the person isn't your husband any
more? Brian isn't just sick or going through a bad patch. He isn't Brian any more. Please
tell me what you think—you are an expert—am I bound by my marriage vows?

Of course, I'm not *that* sort of expert, but Alison requires an answer. She also
requires compassion and support. But all I can think of to say is something
along the lines of doing what she thinks is best, thinking about what the husband
she used to know might have wanted for her, not feeling guilty about considering her own needs, thinking of the welfare of the children, etc. Alison then asks
me another question, 'My husband was a committed Christian. He has no
interest in church or spiritual things now, and he behaves so badly at times.
Will he go to heaven or has he forfeited his salvation?'

Strangely, the answer to this abstract theological question seems quite clear
to me amidst the confusion about how Alison should actually live her life.
I assure her that I believe that his head injury will have made no difference to
her husband's standing in the sight of God. I sincerely believe this to be true,
and anyway I desperately want to provide her with some comfort, to make
things alright. But as soon as the words are out of my mouth I start to wonder
if I have behaved unprofessionally. I am a psychologist not a priest. My own
value system should not intrude into my clinical practice. Or should it?

Alison wearily takes her leave. As she goes out of the door I pause to wonder
what I would do in her situation. I feel like crying myself.

But there is no time to think about her further because I am already late for
the weekly admissions meeting. At this meeting the interdisciplinary team discusses the waiting list for admission for in-patient rehabilitation. Decisions
are reached democratically on the basis of the clinical capacity of the unit and
the needs of the patients on the waiting list. As I enter the room a heated discussion is taking place. The junior doctor has been visiting the trauma ward of
one referring hospital to check on the progress of patients awaiting transfer.
She has got to know the family of one young man who sustained a severe head
injury some weeks previously. She is keen that his admission should be given
priority. But there are several patients ahead of him on the waiting list. She
argues strongly as his advocate, pointing out that he is young, that he has great

potential for rehabilitation, that he is physically and cognitively 'ready' for rehabilitation and if he is not transferred soon his behaviour and physical state may deteriorate. Other team members point out that other patients have been waiting longer for transfer. She replies that it in that case it won't hurt them to wait a bit longer, and their needs are not so urgent. She implies that, as most of them are middle aged, they have had a full life in the past, whereas this young man was on the brink of adulthood when his injury occurred. Surely this is unfair? The rest of the team disagree and decide not to admit him this week. The doctor is clearly upset. Later she tells me that she will have to face that family each time she visits the trauma ward. She feels that as a doctor she should have been able to make a difference to their position. The young man is a university student who reminds her of her own brother. She says she feels let down by the team, powerless, and ashamed because by choosing not to admit him immediately the team is complicit in a deterioration in his physical and mental state. But she wonders if she has got too emotionally involved with this particular family.

The patient at the top of the waiting list is a 60-year-old woman with a history of heavy drinking, who recently had a right hemisphere stroke. She has made a relatively good physical recovery and would therefore have light physical care needs. However, she has gone missing from the referring medical ward several times and been found wandering in the hospital. She says she wants to go home. The occupational therapist has visited her and thinks she would benefit from rehabilitation aimed at improving her safety in self-care and domestic activities, and should be admitted immediately. I ask if the woman has agreed to be transferred to our unit for rehabilitation. The occupational therapist replies that she has definitely not consented, but her insight is poor and she could not be discharged home safely anyway. The two nurses present discuss between themselves whether it would be acceptable to lock part of the ward if she were admitted.

The next patient on the list is a young woman who is very severely physically disabled as the result of an anaesthetic accident. She is due to be admitted from home for a period of assessment. At home her carers help her to smoke by lighting and holding cigarettes for her. Her family has requested that she have the same facility when admitted to the unit. The consultant asks the nurses how they feel about this request. One nurse says she is prepared to discuss it further with her colleagues, the other clearly states her objections on moral grounds, and her refusal to be involved with any care plan that incorporates this practice.

We then discuss two patients who have been referred to the unit, in order to decide whether to accept the referrals and place them on the waiting list. The first of these is a heavy drinker who has for many years been living on the streets, with occasional hostel stays. He has sustained a head injury as the result of an assault by another street drinker. Since admission to hospital his general health condition has improved dramatically. He is well nourished, clean, and has dried out. The team discusses his rehabilitation potential. In the short term he may make a good physical recovery, but in the longer term his social outlook is assessed as bleak. Someone asks if he should be on the waiting list at all. If the actual difference that can be made is likely to be negligible would it be better to use the team's scant resources on more 'appropriate' cases? Another team member angrily asks if we are dividing patients up into the morally 'deserving' and 'undeserving'. Her colleague replies that it is instead a practical question of cost-effective use of limited healthcare resources. I reflect to myself that it is still a question of placing value on an individual's life.

The second new referral is a young man said to be in a minimal awareness state following a severe head injury sustained in a road traffic accident. He is currently cared for in a nursing home but his parents feel he has the potential to improve significantly. The physiotherapist has been to visit him. She reports that he is in a 'vegetative' state, and sees no point in his being put on to the waiting list at all. The consultant, who has met the parents, agrees that chances of improvement are minimal, but says that they need to be given hope, to feel that they can do all that could be done, and there is a genuine chance that the team may be able to effect some small improvements to his care regimen at least. The nurses and physiotherapists counter that such patients make heavy demands of hands-on staff (something that will not affect the consultant) with the inevitable consequence that other patients with less physical care needs will receive less attention. The physiotherapist also asks if it is really fair to the parents to collude with their false hopes in this way.

The meeting concludes with a decision to admit the 60-year-old woman at the top of the waiting list, the one patient we have discussed who definitely does *not* wish to be admitted for rehabilitation. I leave feeling mentally and emotionally tired, and not entirely satisfied that we have arrived at the right outcomes.

Contemporary ethicists may indeed 'entertain theories about human nature, explore the nature of value, discuss competing accounts of the best way to live, ponder the connections between ethics and human psychology, and discuss practical ethical quandaries', but they are not unique in this respect. As this fictionalized but authentic account of an afternoon in a neurological rehabilitation unit I hope makes clear, clinicians involved in the rehabilitation of people with brain injury do this all the time. Clinicians may argue that they are not trained or equipped to wrestle with problems of this degree of philosophical complexity. But at least they have clinical expertise. This puts them in a better position than the family and friends of people with brain injury. These in turn are in a better position than the 'patient', who may also be trying to engage with such questions while experiencing cognitive impairment. (Even Brian is, in his own concrete way, was responding to his perception that all was not right with his marriage by suggesting divorce.)

Yet all three groups, clinicians, families, and people with brain injury themselves, are confronted by what can broadly be described as 'ethical' questions as part of their daily life, with an urgency that does not affect the academic ethicist. In the real world of brain injury rehabilitation decisions have to be taken, and the people who take those decisions have to live with the consequences. The decisions are not just intellectually challenging, they are associated with intense and complex emotions—anxiety, frustration, anger, guilt, shame.

1.2 About this book

This book takes a broad approach to ethics—starting from the position that ethical concerns are essentially concerns to 'do the right thing', and more specifically in this context to 'do the right thing with respect to other persons'. This broad understanding of ethics does not see it as divorced from the rest of life but rather as integral to professional and personal living. For the most part, 'doing the right thing' or 'living the good life' involves habitual behaviour and barely conscious assumptions—'rules for doing the right thing' (for instance trying not to give unnecessary offence to others).

'Doing the right thing' is also part of good technical clinical practice. Clinicians are trained to do the right thing according to the conventional wisdom of their professional bodies. In addition to learning specific techniques, this involves active learning of value systems that underpin the profession's required standards of practice (for instance an emphasis on respecting the confidentiality of patients or promoting their physical independence). This also involves learning the grounds of knowledge (Richards and Bergin 2005) that the profession considers legitimate and the methods that it considers acceptable for evaluating clinical effectiveness (for instance exclusive reliance on large randomized controlled trials). As training proceeds the conventional wisdom that was initially acquired by conscious study becomes part of the clinician's assumptive world. Clinical practice—'doing the right thing with respect to patients' can then proceed in a skilled automatic and streamlined fashion.

From time to time, however, situations arise that challenge personal or professional assumptions and require some conscious deliberation over how to behave

(Wilson 2002). These situations are usually characterized by novelty, complexity, or partial information. Situations of this sort tend to evoke conflict, either within an individual clinician or between colleagues. The conflict may be between different assumptions that had previously appeared compatible. An example from everyday life would be 'always tell the truth' versus 'never intentionally give offence'. An example from clinical practice would be 'do your best to preserve life' versus 'do your best to relieve suffering'. Or the conflict may be between different ways of enacting the same assumption such as telling the truth face to face versus telling it in a letter, or feeding versus administering medication as ways of preserving life.

We recognize such situations by the feelings of anxiety and unease, and the mental perplexity that accompany them (Gaudine and Thorne 2001). Ethical concerns emerge into our consciousness in conflict situations of this sort. So, when we speak about ethics, we are often really referring more specifically to *ethical dilemmas*. Dilemmas have been defined as complex problem situations that involve tension and paradox, where all potential solutions appear to be unfavourable, where potential solutions conflict, and where it is difficult to act (Sekerka *et al.* 2004). What makes a dilemma *ethical* is the intention of the parties involved to 'do the right thing'.

This book is about doing the right thing when faced with the dilemmas that arise in the context of acquired brain injury (ABI). It will be argued that brain injury rehabilitation is a potent and distinctive source of ethical dilemmas because it involves profound novelty, great complexity, only partial information, and a coming together of several different value systems and assumptive worlds (Malec 1993; Tarvydas and Shaw 1996). While some of the ethical issues that arise in the context of ABI also arise in the context of other disabling neurological conditions, such as spinal cord injury, multiple sclerosis, or the dementias, there is a unique combination of factors that applies to ABI. These factors have specific psychosocial consequences, and raise specific ethical issues:

◆ the onset of the condition is sudden in previously healthy individuals
◆ physical, cognitive, emotional, behavioural control systems are all potentially compromised and because of this an unusually large range of professionals may be involved
◆ the outcome is uncertain and improvements may continue for many years
◆ a relatively young population is affected
◆ life expectancy is often normal.

Some of these factors are explored in more depth in Chapter 2. Here it should merely be noted that, although parts of this book may be helpful to practitioners working with people with a wide range of neurological impairments or physical disabilities, its primary focus is the distinctive ethical and psychological challenge posed by brain injury rehabilitation.

The aim of the book is to support all interested parties participating in rehabilitation following brain injury in making good choices in difficult situations, to act effectively on the basis of these choices, and to understand and manage the complex feelings that accompany hard choices and living with uncertainty.

The emphasis is on thinking, action, and feeling because all three are involved in ethical practice. It is important to be able to think through a dilemma clearly and to reach a decision on what constitutes right action. But this is not on its own sufficient for ethical practice. Ethical practice is constrained by what is actually practicable, both in terms of available physical resources and finance (Beauchamp and Childress 2001), and in terms of human psychology (Bersoff 1999). There is a gap between knowing the good and doing the good, and systematic attempts to bridge this gap are an essential part of ethical practice. In addition, because ethical dilemmas can never by their nature be resolved to the complete satisfaction of everyone involved, some acknowledgement must be made of the emotional cost both of the process of decision making and its final outcome.

Thinking, action, and feeling are the province of human psychology, where they are more usually referred to as the domains of cognition, behaviour, and emotion. This book is written by a psychologist, and offers a psychological rather than a philosophical perspective on ethics, engaging with these three domains. It is nevertheless informed by a distinctive philosophy and system of values. These are personal to the author, but have also emerged from experience in clinical practice stretching over many years. They are discussed in more detail in Chapters 3 and 4.

Although the perspective offered is psychological, the intended audience is multiprofessional (and hopefully much of the book will also be accessible to people with no background in healthcare). Brain injury rehabilitation depends on the effective functioning of interdisciplinary teams comprising therapists, doctors, nurses, and others, not least patients and families (McGrath and Davis 1992; Wade 1999). All can be considered 'interested parties' and no single profession has a monopoly on ethical practice. Managing ethical dilemmas in the context of an interdisciplinary team presents special challenges. The potential for conflict is enormous, but so is the potential for mutual support. Managing interdisciplinary conflict and benefiting from interdisciplinary diversity will form a particular focus of this book.

Following this introduction, *Ethical Practice in Brain Injury Rehabilitation* presents a description of ABI and the range and complexity of its consequences in Chapter 2. This aims to give a flavour of what it *feels like* to have a brain injury, and should also form a useful basic introduction for those new to the field of ABI, or fill basic gaps in knowledge for those professionals whose knowledge base is limited to their own speciality. Those readers who are very familiar with the field may wish to skip or skim this chapter. Chapter 3 introduces an approach informed by both neuropsychology and philosophy of mind, explores the notion of brain injury as an assault on personal identity, and argues that person-centred rehabilitation practice flows naturally from this understanding. Chapter 4 presents a discussion of moral values, arguing that person-centred practice is also desirable on moral grounds. Chapter 5 builds on Chapter 4 to give an account of the features of good rehabilitation practice. In Chapter 6 a simple heuristic guide for ethical practice, dealing with thinking, action, and feelings, is presented. This is intended to be user-friendly and applicable to a wide range of situations. Chapter 7 is the final chapter and takes the form of a series of worked cases, each using the heuristic, and each addressing a particular ethical issue. These worked cases have been prepared in consultation with rehabilitation practitioners from a range of disciplines.

I have tried to keep references to a minimum (nevertheless there are many). They only appear in the text to substantiate points that are key to the argument or that are relatively obscure or contentious. Suggestions for further reading are provided at the end of Chapters 2–5.Technical terms are usually explained where they first occur in the text, but there is also a glossary at the end of the book.

Because the issue of being a person is central to this book, every effort is made to refer to individuals with brain injury as 'person' or 'people' throughout. Where this would result in an overly long sentence they are referred to as 'patients' for clarity and conciseness. Terms such as 'patient', 'client', and 'service-user' are all unsatisfactory in their own ways, and the decision to use 'patient' in this book is simply based on personal taste.

Comparable numbers of male and female case examples are presented, and examples in the text are alternately male and female. The examples concerning sexuality and partner relationships are all heterosexual, but can equally be applied to same sex preference and relationships. Unattributed quotes from patients are all drawn from interviews that have been part of research projects into the emotional impact of brain injury, that have received ethical committee approval, and in which the participants have consented to publication of their words.

All case descriptions and names are fictitious, but naturally arise from my clinical experience and that of my sources. If some appear very familiar this is because, despite the uniqueness of each case, there are recurring themes that characterize the aftermath of brain injury. This is good news. Such themes can provide practitioners with a way of ordering complex human issues that might otherwise threaten to overwhelm our mental and emotional resources.

References

Bersoff D (1999). Why good people sometimes do bad things: Motivated reasoning and unethical behaviour. *Personality and Social Psychology Bulletin* **25**, 28–39.

Beauchamp T and Childress J (2001). *Principles of biomedical ethics*, pp. 239–253. Oxford University Press, Oxford.

Gaudine A and Thorne L (2001). Emotion and ethical decision-making in organizations. *Journal of Business Ethics* **31**, 175–187.

LaFollette H (2000). *The Blackwell guide to ethical theory*. Blackwell, Oxford.

Malec J (1993). Ethics in brain injury rehabilitation: existential choices among western cultural beliefs. *Brain Injury* **7**, 383–400.

McGrath J and Davis A (1992). Rehabilitation: Where are we going and how do we get there? *Clinical Rehabilitation* **6**, 255–235.

Richards PS and Bergin A (2005). *A spiritual strategy for counselling and psychotherapy*, pp. 25–69. American Psychological Association, Washington DC.

Sekereka L, Bagozzi R and Jones J (2004). Moral courage in the workplace: self regulation as the cornerstone of virtuous action. *Abstracts of Second European Conference on Positive Psychology*, pp. 153–154. Arcipelago Edizioni, Milan.

Tarvydas V and Shaw L (1996). Interdisciplinary team member perceptions of ethical issues in traumatic brain injury rehabilitation. *NeuroRehabilitation* **6**, 97–111.

Wade D (1999). Goal planning in stroke rehabilitation: Why? *Topics in Stroke Rehabilitation* **6**, 1–7.

Wilson T (2002). *Strangers to ourselves*, pp. 33–35. Belknap Press, Cambridge, MA.

Chapter 2

Acquired brain injury

You treat us like bits and pieces of people.

Lost high up in this enormous hospital in a pink
grey and white unit. Rooms for 'getting bits of
yourself back.' Legs, arms, backs, brains, memory.

This book is about the rehabilitation of people who have acquired brain injury
(ABI) in adulthood. It is therefore important to begin by clarifying the specific
health conditions that are included within this broad term. As noted in the last
chapter, the focus of the book is on acute onset, non-progressive, cerebral
events that arise in the context of previously normal brain function. The
major associated health conditions are closed head injury, stroke, subarachnoid haemorrhage, cerebral hypoxia, and cerebral infections. These health
conditions can be of varying degrees of severity, but the most significant ethical problems are associated with severe conditions. Both the general discussion and the particular case studies in this book concern severe brain injury,
unless specified otherwise.

Different health conditions are associated with different mechanisms that
cause distinctive patterns of brain injury. The effects of deceleration forces
and impact in closed head injury are particularly apparent in certain areas of
the brain. Other brain areas are particularly susceptible to the effects of viruses
or lack of oxygen. Yet other brain areas, defined by cerebral blood supply, are
affected in stroke and subarachnoid haemorrhage. Nevertheless, despite their
differences with respect to cerebral pathology, these health conditions have
much in common. This is because they involve widespread or selective but
strategic brain damage, manifested in multiple psychological and physical
impairments.

The discussion that follows will make use of terminology from the World
Health Organization International Classification of Functioning, Disability
and Health (WHO-ICF) (World Health Organization 2002). This is essentially

a descriptive framework for talking about health conditions at a number of different levels. It is used here primarily to add clarity.[1]

Within the WHO-ICF framework any health condition can be described at three different levels: 'impairment', 'activity limitation', and 'participation restriction'. 'Impairment' is defined as a problem with a body structure and/or body function. 'Activity' is the carrying out of meaningful tasks, and is thus focused on behaviour. 'Participation' is involvement with life situations, and is focused on social role, position, or relationships. Problems at any of these levels occur in, and are affected by personal, physical, and social 'Contextual Factors'.

To give a simplified example, the health condition herpes simplex encephalitis may be expressed at the level of impairment as lesions in the medial temporal lobes of the cerebral cortex (impaired structure) and as anterograde amnesia, the inability to learn new information (impaired function). It may be expressed at the level of activity limitation as a severe difficulty in remembering to keep appointments and pass on messages. It may be expressed at the level of participation restriction as a reduction in employability, with all the associated social disadvantages. Relevant contextual factors are likely to include the previous illness experience and beliefs of the individual (personal context), the availability of prosthetic devices such as electronic memory aids (physical context), and the attitudes of family and potential employers (social context).

In real life, of course, no case is that simple. The problems associated with anterograde amnesia alone extend beyond the area of employment, and a person recovering from herpes simplex encephalitis is anyway likely to have other impairments in addition to anterograde amnesia. The range of possible impairments and, more importantly, possible combinations of impairments, following brain injury is enormous. It is perhaps this that contributes to the feeling of having lost 'bits' of oneself, or having in some sense fallen to bits, expressed by the two patients quoted at the beginning of this chapter.

The more common of these impairments will now be described briefly. For the sake of clarity this will be a greatly simplified account. Impairments can be delineated and classified in various ways. The discussion that follows uses the categories of motor impairment, sensory impairment, visual impairment, auditory impairment, cognitive impairment, and emotional impairment. For each group of impairments common associated activity limitations and psychosocial impacts will be described. (The participation restriction and contextual factors

---

[1] The assumptions underpinning this approach have been questioned by some (see for instance Johnston and Pollard 2001) and its limitations noted (Wade and Halligan 2003), but there is no doubt that it is conceptually clear and descriptively powerful.

that often arise in association with them are considered in Chapter 3 as part of a broader discussion.)

2.1 **Motor impairment**

2.1.1 **Physical basis**

Motor impairment results from damage to brain centres including the motor and pre-motor areas in the frontal lobes of the cerebral cortex, the basal ganglia, and the cerebellum. The type of impairment, and the part of the body affected depend on the extent and location of this damage. Injuries outside the brain (involving the cranial nerves, spinal cord, or the nerve–muscle junctions) can also result in motor impairment. Some patients may sustain motor impairment because of a combination of central brain damage and this other more peripheral damage. This is most common following trauma, for instance a fall or a road traffic accident, which shows no respect for anatomical boundaries. In these cases there may be still further movement difficulties resulting from orthopaedic injuries such as broken limbs.

2.1.2 **Nature of impairments**

Motor impairments can be divided into problems with muscle tone, muscle power, movement coordination, and the presence of unwanted or abnormal movements.

Muscle tone is the level of tension in a muscle that is at rest. There is normally a degree of tension in muscles, higher when a person is alert, lower when she is relaxed or asleep, whose function is to resist the effects of forces acting on the body, such as gravity. Normal tone is a prerequisite for effective movement, and its control is highly complex, involving a number of different brain centres. Tone may be increased or decreased as a result of brain injury; often one group of muscles has increased tone and another group decreased tone in the same patient. Increased tone is expressed in chronically tense or rigid body parts. Decreased tone is more difficult to detect. In severe cases the body parts concerned are 'floppy' like those of a rag doll.

Muscle power refers to the basic strength and weakness in active movement. Following brain injury a patient may actively will a strong movement but only be able to effect a flicker. If no movement at all can be effected it is appropriate to speak of paralysis. Muscle weakness and abnormal muscle tone often occur together because the same or adjacent brain centres and pathways are involved in their control.

Problems with co-ordinating movements ('ataxia') usually arise from damage to the cerebellum and associated pathways. The patient's movements are typically jerky and, as he tries to carry out an action, increasing tremor may be evident.

Tremor of this sort is the most common type of unwanted movement seen following brain injury.

2.2 Sensory impairment

2.2.1 Physical basis

Sensory impairment results from damage at any point in the sensory pathways or in the brain centres concerned with the sensation of pain, touch, temperature, or body position. The sensory pathways begin in receptors in the skin, muscles, joints, and inner ear. They terminate mainly in the thalamus and in the sensory areas in the parietal lobes of the cerebral cortex via spinal nerves and the spinal cord, or directly via the cranial nerves. As in the case of motor impairment, the type of impairment and the part of the body affected depend on the location of the injury. The distribution of the sensory impairment may not be identical with that of the motor impairment in the same patient.

2.2.2 Nature of impairments

On the whole, brain injury results in reduced or absent sensation rather than abnormal sensation. Neurological pain is not a major problem unless the brain injury is compounded by damage to the spinal cord or nerves. Nevertheless, people with ABI may experience significant pain due to complications such as limb contractures or other orthopaedic injuries.

2.2.3 Implications of motor and sensory impairment: activity limitation

Where abnormal tone, weakness, or ataxia affect one or both arms, practical activities such as dressing are very difficult. Where one or both legs are affected walking may be difficult or impossible. Where the muscles associated with speech production are affected articulation difficulty ('dysarthria') results. When faced with these impairments, and the associated activity limitation, patients typically express intense frustration. The effort required to carry out simple movements can be extremely fatiguing. These impairments can lead to socially embarrassing situations, for instance not being able to feed oneself when eating in public, or not being able to make oneself understood to a stranger.

One important movement function that can be affected by brain injury is the ability to swallow. Difficulties with swallowing ('dysphagia') arise when the muscles of the palate and pharynx, or muscles that in turn modulate their activity, lose power and or change tone. This is a common consequence of damage to the brainstem. Patients with dysphagia may be at risk of inhaling food, and thus at risk of choking or developing aspiration pneumonia. Because they cannot swallow their own saliva they may dribble. This condition is managed by careful control of the consistency of the patient's food. Many people with dysphagia exist on a diet of purees and artificially thickened liquids, which they heartily dislike.

Sensation and motor function are underpinned by anatomically distinct (though often adjacent) pathways, and they are also conceptually distinct. Nevertheless normal functional movement is dependent on both systems being intact. Movement is guided by sensory feedback about the position of joints in relation to each other, about the nature of the terrain and one's position in relation to it, about one's position in relation to the midline, and so on.

2.2.4 Implications of motor and sensory impairment: psychosocial impact

Sensory impairment can be experienced as profoundly strange and unpleasant. Limbs affected by significant sensory impairment may feel as if they have been lost or as if they no longer belong to the patient. In rare cases a combination of sensorimotor and cognitive impairment can result in circumscribed delusions, such as 'supernumerary phantom limbs'.

At a more mundane level changed sensation can often lead to a loss of confidence in one's own body and the solidity of the surrounding world. People who have problems walking due to motor impairment or the weakness associated with being very unwell need to be held, physically supported, or lifted as a routine part of their treatment and care. This involves placing trust in the people or equipment doing the lifting and handling. Trust may be stretched to its limits in the absence of the physical sensations that normally indicate being held safely or resting on a solid reliable surface. The presence of pain also makes being lifted and handled a potentially frightening experience.

Learning to walk again may mean relying on a weak limb to bear one's body weight. This is a sufficiently challenging notion in itself, but with the added consideration of absent, attenuated, or distorted sensory signals from that limb it can become a major source of anxiety. Being asked to weight-bear on an affected limb is experienced by many patients as something like being asked to step out into space. It is therefore not surprising that fear of falling can emerge as a significant concern in the context of physical rehabilitation (Friedman *et al.* 2002; Collicutt McGrath 2007). It may also persist in residual form after rehabilitation is completed. Long after they have learnt to walk again many people with weakness or paralysis on one side, who have one essentially normal limb, show a habitual reluctance to weight-bear on the affected side. Here is a description by one physiotherapist of a patient who was

not able to communicate by speech but who showed signs of fear in physiotherapy sessions:

> She avoids standing activities with one on the right (hemiplegic) side. She pulls her-
> self back to sitting. She tries to communicate she is not happy after she has sat down
> in response to 'yes/no' questions. I feel her sensation is poor and she suddenly
> becomes unaware whether her leg is bent or straight in standing.

After consciousness has been regained, the primary concern for most people
with ABI and their families is walking. Physiotherapy directed at independent
walking is very often seen as the core component of the multidisciplinary
rehabilitation programme. There are frequent questions about whether independent walking will be achieved and, if so, how long it will take. Sometimes
patients and their families hold to the belief that walking will be achieved in
the face of information to the contrary provided by rehabilitation professionals.
They may seek out other expert opinions or engage in alternative therapeutic
programmes. Some people who have not walked for many years retain a hope
that they may some day achieve this goal (and indeed some do, see for instance
Keren *et al.* (2001).

What professionals mean by 'walking' and what a patient means by 'walking'
may be very different. When a patient asks if he will walk again he usually has
in mind his pre-injury walking abilities. The professional may have in mind
walking with an unusual gait, wearing an orthotic device to support the ankle,
using a walking aid, and being restricted to short distances on even ground.
Most experienced rehabilitation professionals sense this disparity and do not
confront it directly, tolerating a certain amount of ambiguous discourse in this
area. This is because they are at some level aware that the functional walking
that they have in mind is not just a pale version of what the patient wants, but is
profoundly different. For the patient and her family walking signifies a lot more
than simply getting from A to B independently. It relates, among other things,
to physical appearance and social role, but most importantly it is intimately
connected with a feeling of personal autonomy. There is a sense in which the
question, 'Will I walk again' can be understood to mean, 'Will I be me again?'

In reality 'being me' involves many more things than walking. Unfortunately
these things are also all potentially compromised by brain injury.

2.3 Visual impairment

2.3.1 Physical basis

As with motor and sensory impairment, visual impairment can arise from
damage outside the brain, to the eyes and the optic nerves, or from damage to
the visual pathways and centres in the brain itself. Traumatic injury to the

head may result in a number of visual impairments due to a combination of injuries in some or all of these locations. Within the brain the two areas most important for vision are the lateral geniculate bodies in the thalamus and the visual areas in the occipital lobes of the cerebral cortex, collectively known as 'visual cortex'.

Information from right and left sides of the visual fields of both eyes is carried along independent pathways that cross and re-cross in a complex route to the visual cortex. However, from quite an early stage information from the right visual fields is routed through the left side of the brain and information from the left visual fields is routed through the right side. Therefore, damage to the visual pathways on the right results in difficulty in seeing on the left and vice versa. A range of patterns of visual field loss can occur, depending on the precise location and extent of visual pathway damage.

2.3.2 Nature of impairments

The arrangement of cells in the visual centres of the brain is like a series of maps of the visual fields of the eyes. In the visual cortex each map plots out the visual field in terms of specific physical features of varying complexity such as orientation, colour, and movement. Thus damage to the visual cortex may result in a total loss of vision—'cortical blindness', or a more selective problem in processing aspects of the visual world such as colour.

Centres in the frontal and occipital lobes of the cerebral cortex are concerned with the strategic voluntary control of eye movements so that objects in the environment can be fixated or tracked. Damage to these centres and their associated pathways can result in the patient being unable to reach accurately for static or moving objects.

2.3.3 Activity limitation

The visual difficulties of people with ABI are not always recognized or given the professional attention that they merit. Their practical impact can be enormous. They can result in many problems in activities of daily living that are sometimes wrongly attributed by others to poor cognition.

Difficulties arising from visual impairment can also be compounded by impaired control of the muscles around the eyeballs (that is from motor impairment), resulting in squints and double vision. Unwanted eye movements can also occur, the most common of which is nystagmus, mainly associated with damage to the cerebellum and brain stem. In this condition one or both eyes move to and fro vertically, horizontally, or in rotation.

One major area of activity limitation associated with visual impairment is driving. A significant number of people are excluded from driving following brain injury on the basis of their acquired visual impairment alone. The relationship balance within families can be profoundly changed as the person who was once the main driver is now driven by others:

> My wife drives me and uses little roads because she doesn't like the by-pass, the traffic was bad and it took a long time. I do sometimes feel almost uncontrollably desirous of taking over in driving situations.

2.3.4 Psychosocial impact

Driving has much in common with walking. It signifies and gives real independence and autonomy. For many people their car is almost an extension of their body, and the type of car they drive expresses something of their personality. The personal impact of ceasing to be a driver should not be underestimated.

Learning to walk again is even more challenging if vision is impaired. Being unable to reach accurately is frustrating and can lead to accidents and embarrassment. Unwanted eye movements and squints are disfiguring. Provision of spectacles with corrective lenses may improve function significantly, but spectacles may not be welcomed by the patient because they are seen as unattractive, ageing, and incongruous with self-image. (There is a similar issue with walking aids but these are not 'worn'.) To quote one patient, 'It's bad enough being paralysed without being a specky-four-eyes as well.'

2.4 Auditory impairment

Problems with hearing resulting from brain injury are not as frequently reported and have not been as extensively investigated as problems with vision. Damage to the ear or associated cranial nerves may occur alongside traumatic brain injury. This may result in hearing loss, tinnitus, or vertigo. These symptoms can also arise as a result of brain stem damage. Tinnitus and vertigo are unpleasant symptoms that can be difficult to manage. 'Cortical deafness' has also been reported following damage to the auditory areas in the temporal lobes of the cerebral cortex (auditory cortex).

2.5 Cognitive impairment

The term 'cognition' covers a broad spectrum of mental conditions and activities ranging from simply being alert to engaging in the highest cogitative functions. Impairments in the areas of attention, action, perception, memory, language, executive function, or some combination of these, are to be expected following brain injury. This is because damage to almost any part of the brain has consequences for cognition. Cognitive impairment may resolve fairly quickly for some patients, but the majority experience continuing problems in this area.

2.5.1 **Physical basis**

The relationship between brain function and higher cognition is highly complex and may well vary between individuals. A very simplified summary of the main cognitive impairments and the broad locations of the brain injury thought to underpin each of them are set out in Table 2.1, and a more detailed description follows.

Table 2.1 Summary of the relationship between cognitive impairments and location of brain damage

Type of cognitive impairment	Associated with damage to:
2.5.2(a) Attention—vigilance	Right frontal lobe
2.5.2(b) Attention—general resource	Diffuse brain areas
2.5.2(c) Attention—strategic control	Frontal lobes
2.5.2(d) Attention—orientation to environment	Right parietal lobe, thalamus
2.5.3(a) Visual perception—object knowledge	Temporal lobes and connections with occipital lobes
2.5.3(b) Visual perception—spatial location	Right parietal lobe
2.5.4(a) Action—purposeful organization of movements	Left parietal lobe and its junctions with frontal lobe
2.5.4(b) Action—gesture and object use	Left parietal lobe and its junction with temporal lobe
2.5.5(a) Language—expression	Widely distributed but focused on left inferior frontal lobe
2.5.5(b) Language—comprehension	Widely distributed but focused on junction of left temporal and parietal lobes
2.5.5(c) Language—prosody	Right frontal lobe
2.5.6(a) Memory—storage	Widely distributed cortical areas
2.5.6(b) Memory—automatic encoding and retrieval	Temporal lobes, thalamus
2.5.6(c) Memory—strategic encoding and retrieval	Frontal lobes
2.5.7 Executive function	Frontal lobes

2.5.2 Attention: nature of impairment, activity limitation, and psychosocial impact

A certain level of arousal and alertness is obviously necessary for effective cognition. Even when a previously unconscious patient has regained consciousness he may find that he has lost the simple ability to remain alert over a sustained period (2.5.2(a)). People with this problem may find that they can no longer enjoy reading books or watching long films, or cannot carry out work tasks such as concentrating on a factory conveyer belt to detect faulty products, or proof reading a piece of text.

Attention can be understood as the basic general resource used in cognitive activity. This resource is very often depleted following brain injury as a result of diffuse loss of neurons and their connections (2.5.2(b)). This sort of diffuse damage may occur because of the physical forces causing shearing of the brain in closed head injury. It can also result from biochemical changes secondary to brain injury of any origin. It is expressed psychologically as a general slowness and inefficiency in processing information.

A depleted resource must be carefully managed and deployed. This requires cognitive effort and it is tiring. Cognitive fatigue—a feeling of loss of mental stamina—is a common complaint among people with brain injury (2.5.2(c)). The ability to deploy attention appropriately (to divide it between more than one source, to focus down on one source, to prioritize different demands, etc.) is obviously doubly important in this situation. Unfortunately, this strategic ability may itself also have been compromised. So a depleted resource may be poorly controlled and managed, and the problem is compounded. People with this problem find that they are highly distractible and are no longer able to function effectively in situations that demand multitasking and involve time pressure. Running a home, parenting small children, managing a busy telephone switchboard, serving in a fast food outlet are all examples of such situations. These can become extremely stressful and may lead to emotional responses such as anxiety and irritability, or more physical symptoms such as headache and fatigue.

Finally, the ability to notice and pay attention to objects of significance in the environment, and then to disengage attention appropriately is also crucial for effective cognition. Impairments of this ability can range from a subtle lack of environmental awareness to the more dramatic syndrome of 'neglect' (2.5.2(d)). A person with this problem has great difficulty in disengaging attention from one side of space—usually the right, and may bump into objects on the left, ignore people on the left, physically neglect the left side of her body, only read the left half of a page of print, and so on.

This is a problem over and above any of the visual or sensory difficulties described above. Nevertheless patients often conceptualize it as a problem with eyesight that could be corrected with spectacles. In their turn families and professionals find it very difficult to grasp that constant prompting makes little difference. It can, if anything, become a cause of friction:

> What makes me irritable? Permanent nagging from my family to look to the left.

2.5.3 **Visual perception: nature of impairment, activity limitation and psychological impact**

An intact visual system is necessary but not sufficient for perception of the world. The visual system processes the physical characteristics of the environment, its contours, colours, and so on. But more is required to make sense of the environment. Objects have to be distinguished, identified, and located in space.

Human beings hold a vast quantity of knowledge of objects and their forms and functions, for instance the knowledge that one smooth green spherical object is good to eat and another similar object is something to throw and catch in play. Brain injury can result in loss of access to such knowledge (2.5.3(a)). The patient may stare at an object, be able to describe its physical appearance but unable in any way to indicate what it is.

The technical term for this problem is 'agnosia'. It is important to be clear that this is not a simple problem in naming the object, but a more complex problem in *knowing* the object. It can lead to all sorts of practical problems in the area of self-care and in domestic activities, for instance mistaking bottles of oil or juice for bottles of detergent or bleach, or mistaking the kitchen sink for the lavatory bowl.

A very specific and potentially disabling form of this problem is the inability to identify familiar faces, 'prosopagnosia'. People with this problem may be unable to recognize spouse, parents, or children, with consequent distress to all concerned. Rarely, delusions such as 'Capgras syndrome' may develop.

The location of objects is a distinct psychological process from their identification, and is underpinned by activity in different areas of the brain. Damage to these areas may result in spatial disorientation (2.5.3(b)). A person with this problem may get lost easily, even in familiar environments. This can be a significant problem in hospitals and other communal rehabilitation settings where patients have to find their way to their own bed or bedroom among many others on a ward, or to therapy sessions at some distance. In the longer term, any type of activity beyond the familiar but restricted environment of the home can present a major challenge.

Not feeling securely grounded in the wider environment may lead to a loss of self-confidence, a feeling of always being at a disadvantage. Alongside this, there may emerge a tendency to blame the environment itself, or those managing the environment, for its alienating character. The patient may complain that others have moved landmarks, removed directions, or even reorganized the whole environment. Rarely, delusions such as reduplicative paramnesia may develop.

Problems with visual perception can clearly lead to embarrassing situations. The affected person may appear recalcitrant, forgetful, and difficult. As in the case of visual neglect, patients and their families may conceive of the difficulty as an eyesight problem and request corrective spectacles.

2.5.4 Action: nature of impairment, activity limitation, and psychosocial impact

Intact motor and sensory systems are necessary for normal movement. But action requires more than movement. It requires organized and purposeful movement. It has a major cognitive component that involves spatial and conceptual processing, together with establishing and accessing a repertoire of movement patterns.

For effective action objects in the immediate environment need to be located in relation to body position, and in terms of the movements necessary to reach them. The position of body parts in relation to each other must also be monitored (2.5.4(a)).

In addition there must be knowledge of the action sequences that are typically associated with an object (for instance that a brush should be held in a certain way and operated in a sweeping motion), and 'motor knowledge' (repertoire of familiar sequential movements and postures) (2.5.4(b)).

Damage to the brain centres that are concerned with these abilities and knowledge can result in difficulty in executing purposeful actions even in patients who have no sensory, motor, or other cognitive problems. The technical name for this problem is 'apraxia'. It may affect actions involving one or more limbs or the mouth. People with this problem may have difficulty in walking in a co-ordinated or sustained way, in using objects appropriately (even when they know what they are) or in gesturing, speaking clearly, or writing. They can appear inexplicably clumsy.

It is very difficult either to understand or come to terms with these sorts of difficulties. You know what you want to do. You appear to have all the physical and cognitive capacities necessary to do it. But you can't. The perplexity it evokes is captured by this comment from a doctor following his first examination of a newly admitted patient:

> Having examined her, she performed worse than I would have anticipated at transferring—she didn't seem to know what to do with her legs.

Because of this flavour of 'under-achievement' apraxia can be a major source of frustration and discouragement for all involved, and sometimes of significant performance anxiety for the patient (McGrath 1998).

2.5.5 **Language: nature of impairment, activity limitation, and psychosocial impact**

Whereas speech impairment is essentially a motor problem, impairment of language is a cognitive problem.[2] Language is a hugely complex function and is underpinned by activity in a wide range of locations in the cerebral cortex, and subcortical structures. Both the right and left hemispheres are involved in language function, but injury to the dominant hemisphere (usually the left) is associated with the clearest and most dramatic impairments. Problems with producing and understanding language (dysphasia) are common after left hemisphere stroke because the areas involved in language processing are served by the cerebral blood vessels whose function has been affected by clotting or haemorrhage.

In general damage nearer the front of the dominant hemisphere results in difficulty producing fluent speech (2.5.5(a)), and damage further back results in difficulty in comprehending and producing meaningful speech (2.5.5(b)). However, there is much variability between individuals, and two people with damage to the same part of the brain can have very different types of language impairment.

While damage to large areas of the dominant hemisphere may result in 'global aphasia'—a general and devastating inability to comprehend or produce language of any sort, more circumscribed areas of damage can result in very specific deficits. Careful investigation is required in order to identify and delineate the problem. There may for instance be acquired difficulties in spelling, reading, or naming that only apply to certain categories of word. There may be a specific difficulty in repeating what one has just heard or in writing to dictation. The content of one person's spoken language may be impoverished and full of clichés, the form of another person's language may be restricted and 'telegrammatic'. Again, a person may speak fluently and act as if she understands all that is said to her, using social signals such as nodding and smiling, but on further investigation it may transpire that nothing has been understood. This last type of problem often leads to an overestimation of

---

[2] However, the distinction is not rigid. Disruption of sensorimotor feedback from lips and tongue can have knock-on effects on comprehension, reading, and writing.

abilities by family and rehabilitation staff, and consequent impatience with mistakes. Just as spectacles will not help people who have visual disturbance arising from brain injury, shouting at a person with acquired language impairment will not help (though speaking slowly and clearly might). Unfortunately the experience of people with dysphasia is that quite a lot of shouting goes on.

People who have significant communication problems experience deep frustration. This applies to the mundane practicalities of daily living—difficulty in making telephone calls, reading letters, and talking to strangers all restrict independence. But there is also an enormous impact on relationships with loved ones for obvious reasons. Living with a partner who cannot communicate with you is deeply lonely. There is some evidence that people with significant language comprehension problems following ABI may be at especial risk of developing emotional distress (McGrath 1998), presumably because of a lack of comprehension and control of their environment. Ironically this distress is often missed or left unaddressed because of the very communication problems that caused it in the first place. For instance, people who can only respond to questions cannot initiate requests for help, so everything depends on the right questions being asked in a comprehensible way. It is relatively easy to ask if the person would like a cup of tea. It is hugely effortful to ask if she would like someone to work on her feelings of loss with her (and pointless if someone with the necessary skills is not available).

More subtle changes in language function can also have significant impact on relationships. The non-dominant (usually right) hemisphere is associated with the non-verbal aspects of language—emotional intonation and melodic line of speech (prosody). Just as a person may become unrecognizable after ABI because his gait has changed, he may become unrecognizable because his accent or ability to inject emotion into his speech has changed (2.5.5(c)). One patient recovering from a head injury described sadly how his dog would no longer come to him when he called because he could not produce the intonation that was so familiar to the animal.

2.5.6 Memory: nature of impairment, activity limitation, and psychosocial impact

Remembering an experience or a piece of information involves encoding, storage, and retrieval. Encoding is the process of linking the item to be remembered with existing knowledge. Encoding can take some time, and as it progresses the memory is consolidated, laid down as a strong trace; it is stored. The process of retrieval involves a reactivation of the stored memory.

No single brain centre is concerned with memory storage. Instead, the activity of wide networks of nerve cells all over the cerebral cortex is necessary if different aspects of an episode (the sights, words, smells, thoughts, etc. associated with it) are to be retained. Because these networks are widely distributed it is very rare for memory to be completely wiped out as a result of focal brain injury, although knowledge in certain specific areas may be lost (2.5.6(a)).

In contrast, very specific brain centres are concerned with the *encoding* and *retrieval* of stored memories. As it happens, these areas are particularly vulnerable to the physical shearing and impact forces involved in closed head injury, to some types of infection, and to hypoxia. So memory problems involving encoding and retrieval are extremely common following brain injury. Both encoding and retrieval have an automatic and a strategic component, and we will consider each in turn.

The automatic component relates to the sense of familiarity that is a key component of remembering. Without this automatic encoding and retrieval no new memories can be stored (2.5.6(b)) and the patient will not remember anything that has happened since the brain injury (anterograde amnesia). This is usually a permanent condition, but occurs in temporary form following closed head injury (post-traumatic amnesia). This loss of the ability to remember current information clearly impoverishes mental life. Much of our day-to-day conversation consists of information exchange about current personal or public events. People with anterograde amnesia have great difficulty in this area and it impacts on their ability to sustain relationships. They have a tendency to live in the past. They may ask the same question repeatedly. They forget what they have been told and forget to carry out requested tasks.

The experience of anterograde amnesia has been described as a constant living in the present moment, of carrying out activities, but with no sense of how they relate to a coherent set of life goals. This can lead to a sense of alienation and anxiety:

> You feel as if you were guiding a ship, you feel as if you've lost the steering wheel, and you're shouting at people to go and look after the steering wheel, but you're not sure whether someone is going to do it properly or not. So though you've actually done something, there's this nagging pain in the background that you're not there actually directing it … It totally destroys you.

Sadly, people with anterograde amnesia can still learn to be afraid, even if they do not recall what it is that has made them afraid. This is because the brain centres involved with emotional learning are quite separate from those involved with the learning and retention of declarative information. Thus, anterograde amnesia or post-traumatic amnesia do not protect a person from emotional difficulties such as post-traumatic stress disorder or fear of hospitals (McMillan *et al.* 2003).

Events from long before the injury may be remembered normally. However, because it seems to take some time to lay down strong memory traces, damage to the centres involved in encoding usually also interrupts consolidation, and the patient is consequently unable to remember events hours, days, or even months prior to the injury (retrograde amnesia). This loss of memory of the event leading to the brain injury itself (accident or illness) can be a cause of great distress to both patients and their families. It is a very odd experience to wake up in hospital with no recollection of what has happened to you and to take on trust the explanations of others. Families may have been emotionally traumatized by witnessing or participating in the events that brought their loved-one into hospital. They often communicate their distress to the patient, who is initially perplexed, and later anxious that he will also remember horrific details of what happened to him. Although the period of retrograde amnesia often shrinks, recall of the injury itself is almost unheard of.

As the patient starts to piece together details of what happened, and experiences some return of real memory, he begins to adjust psychologically. Unfortunately this adjustment process may lag weeks or months behind that of his family. This mismatch of the temporal course of adjustment is one significant source of conflict between patient and family. In addition, because the patient may never recollect the early period of his illness he will not be able to empathize with the distress and trauma felt by his family, nor to appreciate the physical care and devotion they may have lavished on him at this time. He may not show the expected level of gratitude, and this can be experienced as deeply hurtful to those who have cared for him.

Occasionally a retrograde amnesia stretching back many years may persist. The patient loses autobiographical memory and memory for public events that happened in the past. This is a tragic state of affairs. A man may not recall his wife of 20 years but remember only his first short-lived marriage. A woman may not recall the birth of her youngest child and thus find it hard to acknowledge that child as her own. The pleasure of personal and communal recollection and nostalgia is no longer available.

Damage to the brain areas concerned with strategic, rather than automatic, encoding, and retrieval result in patchy, confused, and disorganized memory (2.5.6(c)) rather than dense amnesia. Returning to study or to a job where systematic learning is required presents an enormous challenge to a person with this problem. The strategic retrieval of memories involves a kind of active reconstruction. Sometimes irrelevant material, often from the past, is incorporated into an elaborate but essentially false reconstruction (confabulation). People who confabulate can sometimes be misunderstood as liars or fantasists. But they are not making up stories to cover their embarrassment at not remembering.

Rather, because of their cognitive impairments they experience these stories as real memories.

2.5.7 Executive function: nature of impairment, activity limitation, and psychosocial impact

Under normal circumstances human behaviour is closely tied to desired goals. It is strategic. Cognitive abilities function together in an integrated system as the person assesses a situation in relation to a goal, selects a course action to bring it closer to that goal, initiates action, monitors progress toward the goal, and terminates action when the goal has been achieved. The goal may be simple, such as making a cup of tea, or complex, such as planning a wedding reception. In normal life a number of goal-directed projects are always carried out alongside each other, and prioritization is required.

Executive impairment is essentially thinking that has become dislocated from its goals in various respects. People with this group of problems may find it difficult to generate any ideas or strategies at all, or the ideas they do initiate may be very limited. They may have great difficulty in seeing a problem from more than one point of view, often their own. Conversely, they may have no problem in generating ideas and strategies, but these may have little relation to the goal in question, being instead a reaction to something in their immediate environment, or they may begin a promising line of thought but abandon it without reference to their goal. This can give their thinking an impulsive or distracted quality. Finally, they may continue with a train of thought, or repeat a previous train of thought, even when it is clearly inappropriate to their goal. These problems with initiation of ideas, conceptual rigidity, impulsivity, and perseveration are characteristic of executive impairment. All of these thinking styles can also be expressed in behaviour.

While executive problems are seen in their purest form in thinking directed at solving complex problems, they are also evident in the self-regulation of cognitive systems and behaviour. As discussed in some earlier sections, the strategic allocation of attention, the strategic planning of action sequences, the strategic encoding and retrieval of memories, and the seamless integration of cognitive systems, can all be compromised as a result of executive impairment.

Even if all other abilities are intact (and this would be a very rare situation) executive impairment can have devastating effects. Good executive abilities are needed to negotiate the complex, demanding, and nuanced world of social relationships. People with executive impairments are often disorganized but may also appear to have lost spontaneity and humour. Or they may develop a more facile type of humour. Their difficulty in initiating thought and action may look like laziness. Their difficulty in seeing the point of view of others may look like selfishness. Their impulsivity may result in bad decisions. Their difficulty in monitoring their own behavioural strategies may result in an over-optimistic appraisal of their situation.

While all types of impairment following brain injury have the capacity to render the patient less recognizable to others as their old selves, executive impairment is by far the most significant in this respect. Much has been written about how people with these problems appear to others, yet there is relatively little information on what it feels like to live with executive impairment from the perspective of the patient, and the degree to which such patients are less recognizable to themselves. Some types of executive impairment may be closely linked with an impoverished emotional experience (Hornak *et al.* 2003). These people often come over as perplexed, defensive, or unconcerned. This is probably because their ability to self-monitor and to reflect accurately on experience has been compromised. Where poor self-monitoring of this sort is combined with impairments of perception or attention more distinctive difficulties with aspects of self-awareness can result (Clare 2004).

Because these patients may have little in the way of physical disabilities, and give an appearance of normal or even high intelligence, their behaviour is rarely excused by others, but rather attributed to characterological defects.

2.6 **Emotional impairment**

The large range of impairments described above and their consequent limitation of activity clearly have a very significant emotional impact on patients, friends, and families. However, primary impairments in the neurological systems concerned with emotion may also occur following brain injury. For instance, depression is fairly common after brain injury. While this may arise as part of a psychological reaction to illness and injury, there is some evidence that brain changes may make these patients more susceptible to depression (Fleminger *et al.* 2003).

Emotionalism is an increased readiness to cry, or more rarely to laugh usually in emotional situations. People with this problem may weep when shown kindness, when watching sentimental films, or when thoughts turn to loved ones. Laughter may occur in very sad situations such as funerals. The weeping may be profuse and uncontrollable. This is highly embarrassing, especially so for men. It is distressing to witness because the quality of the weeping is redolent of deep anguish. In fact the person may merely be feeling a little 'emotional'. The physical expression of emotion has become uninhibited. People with this problem can become very socially isolated. Few people wish to converse with someone who may burst into tears at any moment. Emotionalism can arise from damage to a number of different centres throughout the brain.

'Alexithymia' is more unusual, and essentially refers to a converse group of problems. These include difficulty in identifying or describing emotional feelings, which can arise because of disrupted connections between the right and left cerebral hemispheres, and a loss or impoverishment of affective experience, which can arise because of damage to the limbic system and its connections with other brain areas. People with these problems can appear detached and shallow. It is extremely hard to maintain a relationship with someone who no longer feels or expresses emotions, and therefore cannot share the emotional experiences, such as joy or grief, of those close to him.

2.7 The total impact of multiple impairments

Some of the impairments described above are relatively simple to understand and explain. Others are conceptually challenging. Some are painful to experience, some are confusing, some embarrassing, some terrifying. In combination they have the potential to be devastating. Learning to walk again might be manageable if your memory hadn't become so bad that you couldn't recall your physiotherapy instructions. Building a relationship with the child you had forgotten might be achievable if you didn't keep bursting into tears when talking to her. Managing your feelings of depression might be possible if only you could get out of your wheelchair and go for a good run. On top of all this people with ABI may be struggling with the effects of medical complications, such as post-traumatic epilepsy, infections, or hydrocephalus.

Combinations of cognitive physical and emotional impairment, together with situational factors, can also give rise to unwanted behavioural change. For instance a woman experiencing cognitive overload arising from impaired attention may respond by becoming irritable, and express this in verbal or physical aggression because the executive system that would normally monitor and control her behaviour has also been impaired. Or a young man who is sexually frustrated because he is hospitalized may masturbate in public because he has neither the physical ability to remove himself to a private space, nor the cognitive abilities first to see that others would be offended by his behaviour, and then to modify his behaviour accordingly.

Life ceases to be a seamless series of integrated, automatic, and balanced behaviours that can be taken for granted but becomes fragmented, effortful, and full of mistakes:

> It's really horrible—a totally new feeling. I feel like a totally different person—I'm not me any more I'm someone else. At times I feel I can step away from myself and watch myself doing something—and I'm doing it wrong. When you're not in charge of your emotions—not in charge of yourself, life is just one big fight—you fight for everything.

For this patient at least, one major effect of the impairments that arose from her brain injury was that she no longer felt like herself. She experienced herself as a different person altogether. In the next chapter we will begin to explore the relationship between brain injury and personal identity more systematically.

Suggestions for further reading

The texts below have been chosen because they convey the experience of living with impairments that arise from brain injury.

Damasio A (1995). *Descartes' error*, Chapters 1–3, pp. 3–51. Papermac, London.

Halligan P and Marshall J (1997). The art of neglect. *Lancet* **350**, 139–140.

Parr S, Byng S and Gilpin S (1997). *Talking about aphasia: living with loss of language after stroke.* Open University Press, Buckingham.

Sacks O (1998). *The man who mistook his wife for a hat and other clinical tales.* Simon and Schuster, New York.

Schachter D (1996). *Searching for memory: the brain, the mind, and the past.* Basic Books, New York.

Solms M and Turnbull O (2002). *The brain, the mind, and the inner world.* Karnac, London.

Wilson B (1999). *Case studies in neuropsychological rehabilitation.* Oxford University Press, New York.

The following are general textbooks that describe neurological impairments in more detail

Basso A (2003). *Aphasia and its therapy.* Oxford University Press, New York.

Kolb B and Wishaw I (2003). *Fundamentals of human neuropsychology.* Freeman, New York.

Stokes M (1998). *Neurological physiotherapy.* Mosby, London.

References

Clare L (2004). The construction of awareness in early-stage Alzheimer's disease: a review of concepts and models. *British Journal of Clinical Psychology* **4**, 155–175.

Collicutt McGrath J (2007). Fear of falling after brain injury. Submitted to *Clinical Rehabilitation.*

Fleminger S, Oliver D, Williams WH and Evans J (2003). The neuropsychiatry of depression after brain injury. *Neuropsychological Rehabilitation* **13**, 65–87.

Friedman S, Munoz B, West S, Rubin G and Fried L (2002). Falls and fear of falling: Which comes first? *Journal of the American Geriatric Society* **50**, 1329–1335.

Hornak J, Bramham J, Rolls E, Morris G, O'Doherty J, Bullock P and Polkey C (2003). Changes in emotion after circumscribed surgical lesions of the orbitofrontal and cingulated cortex. *Brain* **126**, 1691–1712.

Johnston M and Pollard B (2001). Consequences of disease: testing the WHO International Classification of Impairments, Disabilities and Handicaps (ICIDH) model. *Social Science and Medicine* **51**, 1261–1273.

Keren O, Reznik R and Groswasser Z (2001). Combined motor disturbances following severe traumatic brain injury: an integrative long-term treatment approach. *Brain Injury* **15**, 633–638.

McGrath J (1998). *Fear following brain injury*. PhD thesis, Oxford Brookes University.

McMillan T, Williams HW and Bryant R (2003). Post-traumatic stress disorder and traumatic brain injury: A review of causal mechanisms, assessment, and treatment. *Neuropsychological Rehabilitation* **13**, 149–164.

Wade D and Halligan P (2003). New wine in old bottles: the WHO ICF as an explanatory model of human behaviour. *Clinical Rehabilitation* **17**, 349–354.

World Health Organization (2002). *Towards a common language for functioning, disability and health ICF*. World Health Organization, Geneva.

Chapter 3

The person at the centre of rehabilitation

Human psychological universals are core mental attributes shared ... by all or nearly all *non-brain damaged* adult human beings across cultures.

Norenzayan and Heine (2005, p. 763—my italics)

The last chapter was concluded with the idea that acquired brain injury (ABI) is, above all, an assault on the personal. We will now explore this idea in more detail by considering two questions. First, what it is that renders us persons; secondly what it is that renders us human persons. If ethics is about doing the right thing with respect to other persons, it is important to understand how ABI has the potential to rob the individual of recognizable human personal characteristics, so that he may seem to fall outside the scope of ethics altogether. We can slip into unethical practice when dealing with people recovering from ABI simply because we do not perceive them as fully human persons.

A third question will then be considered. What is it that renders us distinctive *individual* human persons? ABI has implications for individual identity that give rise to many ethical dilemmas.

3.1 Being a person

Humans have much in common with other animals, but also share some features of plants and complex computational machines. Although we may talk gently to our plants and shout in frustration at our computers, we do not generally consider these to be persons. In contrast we may do these things to our cat or dog, and genuinely feel that these animals have personal attributes. This is essentially because they are sentient, can respond to us, or even initiate action directed towards us. In addition they appear to have emotions. Emotion is the 'glue' of social bonds, and social bonds involving empathy seem to be important in our experience of others as persons. Persons are feeling entities like us. (This is why doing the right thing with respect to animals is an important area of ethics.)

Some individuals have great difficulty in forming relationships with others, appearing to lack empathy, and failing to display appropriate emotion in social encounters. People with autistic spectrum disorders evident since childhood may fall into this category. Some people with ABI seem to acquire this difficulty too (see for instance Happe *et al.* 1999; Langdon 2003, pp. 243–245). They may also show rigid, inflexible behaviour that has a 'programmed' quality to it. It is not uncommon to come across the language of 'automaton', 'robot', or 'android' in colloquial references to these people or their behaviour. The use of such language indicates that in some sense the individual is seen as falling short of what is required in order to be considered a person.

More dramatically, profound brain injury can result in states of minimal awareness and responsiveness. The individual is apparently no longer sentient. It is not surprising that plant vocabulary, such as 'vegetative state' is invoked to describe such people. Individuals who are not sentient, and show no capacity to become sentient in the future essentially cease to be persons.

3.2 Being a human person

Human beings are like animals and plants, but unlike machines, in that we are biological creatures with our own physiology. On the other hand, like animals and machines, but unlike plants, we engage in complex behaviour, acting on our environment. Moreover we are agents of our behaviour, not requiring specific and detailed programmed instructions in order to initiate actions, and in this respect we are clearly more like animals than machines.

Within the animal kingdom human beings form a biologically distinct species. We can be distinguished from other animals most clearly by our physical form, by our characteristic behaviours (for instance walking upright on two legs, and speaking) and our cognitive abilities. Where the appearance or behaviour of human beings is anomalous, animal vocabulary may be invoked, implicitly raising questions about their human status.

Physical deformities are often described in animal terms, for instance 'buffalo-hump', 'ape-foot', 'bat-ear'. In severe cases of deformity the person himself may be described in animal terms, for instance 'Elephant man'. Where a baby of extremely unusual physical form is born it is not uncommon to hear the word 'monster' whispered. Other terms such as 'dwarf' are less redolent of the animal kingdom, but have definite non-human overtones. In some societies, most obviously Nazi Germany and South Africa under the Apartheid regime, relatively small variants in form due to racial differences have been treated as evidence for the 'subhuman' nature of some groups.

In her book *My Life my Hands* Alison Lapper, who has the condition phocomelia, describes incidents from her early life. Both vegetable and animal vocabulary crop up:

> Can you hear that screaming down the corridor? That's a baby that's just been born. She's got no arms or legs ... The nurses say she'll die in a day or two , or else be a cabbage for the rest of her life ... I expect [the doctors] are waiting for it to die.
>
> We were about 250 children with a variety of impairments ... The staff called us the 'strange little creatures'.
>
> (pp. 13, 20)

Animal vocabulary is also used to describe individuals who engage in behaviour traditionally associated with non-human animals, especially uninhibited aggressive or sexual behaviour. In the tabloid press the terms 'paedophile' and 'beast' are used interchangeably, with the implication that individuals who sexually abuse children have forfeited any claim to being human. In some very conservative African cultures this attitude also applies to homosexuality. The key issue here seems to be that an individual who cannot master his 'lower' desires, but is instead enslaved to them, is seen as less like a human being and more like an animal. This is highly relevant to the situation of people with ABI, especially individuals with significant executive impairment arising from frontal lobe damage. Many of these people experience a loss of inhibition affecting a wide range of behaviours, which can include sexual or aggressive behaviour. These are underpinned by activity in centres that are both anatomically deep down in the brain, and phylogenetically primitive. So there is a biological as well as a moral sense in which such behaviours arise from 'lower' impulses. This is *not* to say that brain injury turns people into sex offenders. (The evidence suggests that this may emerge as a problem for only a small minority; Simpson *et al.* 1999.) However, brain injury can result in a loss of mastery of 'lower' desires that may suggest a falling short of the fully human.

The cognitive abilities of humans far outstrip those of other animals. One way that this is expressed is in the use of past experience to inform intentions for the future, which themselves influence action. This capacity, while arguably present in a rudimentary form in some other animals, is closely related to the emergence of language, and most fully developed in humans. Humans are probably unique in their capacity for self-reflection, itself closely linked with language and intentional thought:

> A non-human animal can feel sensations, perceive things, feel emotions, want things, and act in pursuit of what it wants. It can know a variety of things, and, in a rudimentary

sense, it may think or believe various things. It is, as we are, either conscious or unconscious; ... Nevertheless, it is not a self-conscious creature. It can perceive, but it cannot think about or reflect on the fact that it is perceiving ... Nor can it reflect on its past experience, even though its past experience may affect its current behaviour and actions.

Bennett and Hacker (2003, p. 346)

In summary then, we recognize an individual as a person and a member of the human race if he:

+ is sentient (also true of most animals)
+ can make emotionally nuanced social relationships (also true of some animals)
+ looks human
+ engages in typical human behaviours, such as walking upright and speaking
+ appears to be the controlling agent of his own behaviour
+ shows evidence of some inner mental life expressed as a coherent account of himself

This is also how we recognize ourselves as human persons.

While many physical and mental health conditions may affect some of these human identifying markers, only neurological conditions involving the brain have the capacity to rob the individual of any or all of them. It has already been noted that people in minimal awareness states are thought to lack sentience. It was also observed in Chapter 2 that many people with ABI have difficulty in maintaining social relationships, often because of poor awareness of their own behaviour, or a difficulty in reading the behaviour of others. The motor impairments described in Chapter 2 may result in physical deformities. They may also render an individual capable of merely crawling rather than walking, or of emitting incomprehensible noises rather than recognizable speech. Language impairment may make any communication effectively impossible. Earlier in this section we noted the way in which executive impairment seems to place some individuals at the mercy of their passions. But executive impairment also interferes with thinking, as we saw in Chapter 2. Along with problems with memory and language processing, executive impairment has the capacity to interfere with coherent thinking and self-reflection.

In all these ways the status of individuals as human persons is deeply challenged by ABI. Of course people with conditions affecting the brain are technically biologically human, they still have human DNA. But in other respects they may not seem entirely human, either to themselves or to those around them. They may feel less than human, strange, or different. Not feeling human is a very bad place to be, expressed in the language of informal advance directives as, 'If I become a vegetable turn of the machines!', in the words of one ABI patient as, 'I'm no longer a man—I'm a spaz', and in the words of the psalmist:

> But I am a worm, and not human;
> Scorned by others, and despised by the people.

Psalm 22.6 (New Revised Standard Version)

This last quote refers to one final identifying marker: we recognize an individual as human by the way others behave towards him.

This is because the notion of 'human being' is to an extent socially constructed, as the unhappy quote at the beginning of this chapter makes clear. Some people treat their children like animals, others treat their pets like human beings. Certain types of treatment directed towards prisoners can be aimed at 'dehumanizing' them. This reflects the fact that an individual's humanity is as much ascribed to her by others as it is intrinsic to her nature.

This is the one human identifying marker that is not directly affected by brain injury. The direct effects of brain injury are multiple impairments. As we have seen, by their nature these impairments almost inevitably dehumanize. Managing the effects of brain injury therefore involves managing its dehumanizing effects. This may mean treating certain impairments directly. There is, for instance, a sense in which improving range of movement in limbs, building up strength and balance, and thus re-establishing walking ability renders a patient more fully a human person. And of course, this is one of the factors that lie behind the very strong desire of ABI patients to walk again, discussed in Chapter 2.

But treatment of impairments and their associated activity limitations is not the primary way to address the dehumanizing effects of brain injury. The place to start is treatment of the *person* with the brain injury. Behaving towards people whose humanity is threatened or damaged as if they were fully human actually renders them more fully human in their own eyes, in the eyes of others, and in our eyes. Acknowledging the potential loss of humanity wrought by brain injury and repudiating it through an assertion of the continuing humanity of the individual is understood in this book to be a starting point for ethical rehabilitation practice. It is simply to affirm by word and action that people with ABI fall within the scope of human ethics. Treating impairments arises from this and must always be seen in relation to it. Good technical practice flows from the correct ethical perspective.

Practice principle 1. Despite some appearances to the contrary, people with ABI are human persons and should be treated as such.

What does it mean to treat a patient like a human person? It means behaving towards him as if he has human attributes, and establishing conditions under which these attributes can be expressed, if only in an attenuated form.

At the most basic level this involves:

- attributing sentience and coherent mental life to the patient, even where these are in doubt
- treating the patient's body parts as essential aspects of a whole human being rather than pieces of meat, even when they appear deformed or unresponsive
- supporting the expression of the patient's agency, especially where it is very limited by physical or cognitive impairment
- treating the patient as a social being by making a relationship with him and encouraging others to do likewise.

This appears to be simple good practice, but it is by no means universal practice in interactions with patients, despite good intentions, because the basic assumption of common humanity has somewhere got lost. This is well illustrated by the following quotes from two women with ABI. The first recounts some of her experiences following her admission to hospital. She was conscious but unable to move at all or to communicate due to a brainstem stroke.

> One nurse said, 'She looks dead', which did not do my morale any good at all.
>
> Often lots of people in white coats gathered around, always talking about me and not to me. Some of it was familiar and then they drifted off discussing things I'd never heard of before. I wanted to ask them where I was and why? What they were talking about? How dare they talk as if I was not there! I felt livid, but couldn't get it across.
>
> All my dreadful thoughts and confused state could have been prevented if only the hospital staff had told me what they were doing, even if there appeared to be no response from me. Nobody even explained what had happened to me …
>
> There was a registrar from … [the] rehabilitation centre. I can remember the first time he came to visit me at … Hospital. He actually *spoke* to me. He asked me if I would like the nasal feed tube, which I hated, replaced by a tube in the stomach. I opened my eyes wide and smiled to say yes. It was the first time I remember anyone asking *me* a question about my care.
>
> Quoted by Moore (2003, pp. 69, 72, 73)

The second woman, describes her experience of care at the hands of one nurse when she was in the early stages of recovery following a stroke:

> She manhandled me one morning, transferring me from my bed to my wheelchair by grabbing the back of my pajamas and pulling them up tight to work as a hoisting mechanism. I'd vaguely complained to be told in no uncertain terms that she worked nights. It was not her job to know how to transfer patients who were paralysed.
>
> From *An Abnormal Reality* by Jan Quinlan, unpublished manuscript.

For these women the dehumanizing effects of their brain injuries were magnified by the treatment meted out to them by some healthcare professionals. They were at times treated like objects, acted upon but otherwise ignored.

Now of course, many people with health conditions or physical disabilities that do not involve brain injury sadly also undergo experiences of this sort. But it is illuminating to note some typical indignant reactions to the lack of respect shown to people with physical disabilities:

> Just because someone is deaf, they are not stupid and deserve to be treated with courtesy and respect (Zazove quoted by Rafferty 2003).
> This isn't only a legal issue. It's one of basic respect for the individual. Individuals with disabilities are a part of 'We The People', and as such are entitled to human respect and an opportunity for self-development. From 'My brain works … my legs don't! Let's take the "dis" out of disabilities' (Skinner 2000).

The first quote rightly states that a person with a sensory impairment is entitled to courtesy and respect, but implies that a person with a cognitive impairment may not have such an entitlement. The second quote rightly emphasizes the fact that people with physical disabilities are part of the human race, but the title of the paper implies that this status is dependent on a fully functioning brain.

These attitudes reflect three deeply held assumptions. The first two have been prevalent in western society since the eighteenth century Age of Enlightenment, and are particularly associated with the philosopher René Descartes. The third has emerged more recently with the development of neurology over the last century. All are philosophically suspect.

- the mind and the body are separate entities
- the mind, the thinking faculty, is the essence of the human soul
- the mind and the brain are identical.

So a damaged brain is understood to imply a damaged soul, a partial or complete loss of what makes us human persons. While this understanding can form the basis of a positive therapeutic approach for people with brain injury (Prigatano 1991), its negative side is an implicit questioning of their entitlement to be treated as human persons.

Yet even as we assert that a patient with ABI is a human person, another question, loaded with ethical implications, presents itself. Who is this person?

3.3 **Being me**

As we have seen, brain injury can rob people of features that signify belonging to the human race, but it also affects the things that have, up until the injury, made them distinctive individuals within the human race. It is important to belong to a group but it is also important to know one's place within the group, to know both that you have much in common with others and that you are special and unique. This sense of uniqueness is achieved through the almost infinite variation that is possible within the boundaries of what is deemed 'normal' in relation to human appearance and behaviour.

Brain injury threatens this sense of individuality in two ways. First, the person can lose a whole range of individuating characteristics, so that he appears very different from before. Secondly, some impairments can make an individual appear so like others with the same impairment that it is hard to see him as distinctive. (For instance, people with ataxic dysarthria, speaking in an effortful disjointed monotone, tend to sound the same as each other and different from everybody else.)

This loss of individuating characteristics is a feature of neurological conditions such as Parkinson's disease, Alzheimer's disease, chronic-progressive multiple sclerosis, and so on. The difference in the case of ABI is that the change is sudden and quantal rather than gradual and incremental. Thus the rate of adjustment required of the patient and family is phenomenally quick. This is true even in cases where there has been a long limbo period during which the person with ABI was unconscious, because the usual expectation or hope of relatives and friends is that she will wake up as if from sleep, essentially the same person as she was before. They are therefore psychologically unprepared for major changes in their loved one when she finally regains consciousness.

It can seem as if the previous person has been lost and replaced by a new person overnight. Both the person with ABI and her relatives or friends may experience the situation as a personal change. However they will be viewing it from very different perspectives and may not always agree. It is not uncommon for a patient with ABI to insist that they are the same person 'inside' despite lost abilities, emotional changes, and altered appearance (Collicutt McGrath 2007b), whereas those close to her may experience a profoundly changed person (Oddy 1995).

Certain personal features seem to be treated as essential identity markers by others. Note, for instance, this comment made by the husband of Abigail Witchalls, who sustained a spinal cord injury as the result of a knife attack.

> Benoit Witchalls said: 'She is a remarkable character ... I think I've had a crash course in spinal injury, and you just can't tell anything for the first month, so it's a case of wait and see, really. But she has still got her smile, which is very comforting to see ... We feel very lucky and very blessed because she is fully present as herself. It's just great to see and it's a great joy you can see in her face when she sees Joseph.'
>
> Interview for BBC Crimewatch programme (18 May 2005)

At first glance this seems to be a focus on the mental, psychological, or perhaps even the spiritual, in the context of great physical losses. And yet the things that this husband mentions as indicating the continuing presence of his wife 'as herself' are her familiar smile and facial expression—*physical* actions, taken to signify something beyond them. There is a sense in which if she had no longer been able to smile she would have been experienced by those who love her as less fully 'present as herself'.

This illustrates well the integrated rather than dichotomous nature of the physical and psychological, the practical impossibility of drawing a dividing line between body and mind when talking about real people. Cognitive neuroscientists are increasingly recognizing this to be the case, as they have come to understand that the historical tendency to draw a rigid a distinction between thinking or perception and action has resulted in misleading conclusions about human psychology. Our perception of the world is itself highly influenced by the way we habitually act upon it. Our environment is primarily a place we inhabit rather than a place we observe from somewhere else. Perception is enactive, cognition is embodied (see for instance Varela *et al.* 1991; Hurley 1998; Ginsburg 1999).

In turning to a consideration of the characteristics that make human beings individuals, and that are so often affected by brain injury, we therefore begin with the body. The sections that follow explore the things that enable people to be fully present as themselves, both in their own experience and the experience of those around them.

3.3.1 **Physical identity and integrity**

Individuals resemble other members of their ethnic groups and biological families, but have distinctive facial features, bodily size, relative bodily proportions, and so on. Physical morphology confers both belonging and distinctiveness.

Morphological changes, for instance contractures or weight gain, may arise indirectly from brain injury. The appearance of facial features may change as the direct result of neurological impairments such as weakness in facial muscles, squints, or nystagmus. Surgery or trauma may leave permanent visible scars. A person who can no longer stand upright is effectively diminished in physical height. These sorts of changes make a person less like himself and less like those he used to resemble. He becomes distinctive in a new and unwelcome way.

Individuals are also distinguished from others by the boundary of their bodies and the immediate personal space surrounding it (Geertz 1984). The act of touching or embracing another has the potential to compromise her identity by melding it with that of the other person, and as such most societies have very clear rules of engagement surrounding greetings and embrace (Gurevitch 1989, 1990).

Any sort of serious physical disability or illness means that the person needs to receive some aspects of intimate physical care from others. This may even include entry into orifices, the gateways of the body (Douglas 1966). The boundaries between the body and its physical environment, between the patient and his carers, become blurred. Physical privacy is lost and physical intimacy no longer signifies emotional intimacy.

3.3.2 Free and independent movement and action (autonomy)

A person is also distinct from other people in so far as she, rather than someone else, is the agent of her own behaviour. At the most basic level this means being able to move your arms and legs under your own volition. If your limbs can only be moved by others you take on some of the characteristics of a doll or puppet. This is another personal boundary infringement. Difficulty with movement also hugely restricts the behavioural options available to a person.

Hilary Lister, paralysed for several years by a progressive neurological condition, describes sailing single-handedly across the English Channel:

> It was as if I was flying, that's the only way I have to describe it ... I was free, free, free—for the first time since I can remember. I can't tell you how wonderful it was. I was in charge I had the freedom to say 'I think I'll turn here now.' ... I was in control of my own life and I'd forgotten what that feels like.
>
> *Daily Mail* 27 August 2005

However, difficulty with movement is only one obstacle to the independent enactment of intentions. This also requires the ability to form an intention, work out how to achieve it, remember it, organize the required movements, check progress towards the goal, and so on. Thus, several of the cognitive impairments described in Chapter 2 interfere significantly with effective independent action. They have the effect of diminishing agency. (Note the reference to not having control of the steering wheel of life quoted in Chapter 2.) A person who requires prompts to initiate actions, or scripts to carry them out, is no longer their sole author.

There is, of course a longstanding and unresolved philosophical debate as to whether any decision that a human being makes can truly be said to be free. Nevertheless it is generally agreed that we can distinguish between decisions that *feel* free and spontaneous and those that feel coerced, and we can make similar judgements about the decisions made by other people. We also associate freedom (and responsibility) with choosing between a manageable number of options, as opposed to accepting the only option available.

Autonomy requires agency, and people with ABI are therefore generally less able to make autonomous choices. Autonomy also requires liberty, freedom from coercion. People with ABI are also less able to make autonomous choices because their liberty is often restricted by their physical and social context. In terms of the WHO-ICF model discussed on page 12, their autonomy is compromised because of both impairment (loss of agency) and contextual factors (loss of liberty).

Prisoners, school children, parents with small children, people in debt or with low incomes, and people from stigmatized minority groups all have limited autonomy because their liberty is restricted. None of us has absolute freedom from social restrictions. But people recovering from ABI can face restrictions in a particularly wide range of social and physical areas. They are likely to lose income. They become patients, a word with the same linguistic root as 'passive'. They may become short- or long-term residents of institutions, and be expected to comply with the rules of such institutions (for example, eating all meals with others at a table instead of alone in front of the television). If their mobility is reduced they will find themselves unable to access many buildings, modes of transport, or public places. If they can no longer speak clearly they may need an advocate to speak on their behalf. If they have cognitive problems they may be deemed incapable of making certain decisions, and these may then be taken for them, for instance by the Court of Protection under the Mental Capacity Act (2005).[1] In extreme circumstances they may be regarded as a danger to themselves or others and be detained or treated under Section of the Mental Health Act (1983).[2]

3.3.3 Habitual behaviours and behavioural style

We recognize an individual by the way he carries out actions, for instance by his gait or handwriting. Indeed the way that a person writes his name is described as his 'signature'—a sign of his nature. Any impairment that affects the ability to write removes this formally recognized identity marker.

One philosopher has argued that habitual dispositions or tendencies 'constitute the self' (Dewey 1922/2002, p. 25). We certainly make judgements about people based on their habitual behaviours and behavioural style. For instance

---

[1] The Mental Capacity Act applies to England and Wales. The Scottish equivalent is the 2000 Adults with Incapacity (Scotland) Act.

[2] The 1983 Mental Health Act (England and Wales) is currently under revision. An 'amending bill' will shortly be put before Parliament. The Scottish equivalent is the 2003 Mental Health (Care and Treatment) (Scotland) Act.

we may know that a friend of ours plays a lot of cricket, always leaves things to the last minute, tends to interrupt his conversation partners, and smiles a lot. Another friend may keep her home tidy, read a lot of difficult books, work long hours, and take work home with her. From this we may infer that our first friend is a disorganized extravert who likes cricket, and that our second friend is an intelligent organized workaholic. We construct a picture of their temperaments, abilities, and preferences. Such constructions may be arrived at in collaboration with other friends, and indeed with the person in question. What began as provisional hypotheses to describe behaviour tend to develop into consensual fixed descriptions of 'personality'.

Brain injury deconstructs personality because it removes the ability or opportunity to carry out the behaviours that formed the basis of its construction. (In terms of the WHO-ICF model this is one of the effects of activity limitation.) We will see our friend very differently if he speaks slowly, no longer plays cricket, and never seems to smile. Alongside this he may also experience subjective emotional changes such as deep sadness. He too may see himself differently, though this is less certain.

A particularly helpful way of understanding the behaviour of individuals is in relation to personal goals (Emmons 1999). An apparently random collection of unrelated habitual behaviours may achieve coherence if seen in the light of personal goals. These goals are variously described by psychologists as 'current concerns', 'life tasks', 'personal projects', and 'personal strivings'. Mundane habitual goals, such as getting the grocery shopping done, are thought to be connected to more fundamental goals, often expressed in terms of values related to personal identity, such as being a good mother (Carver and Scheirer 1990; Sheldon and Kasser 1995; McGrath and Adams 1999).

Following ABI the immediate goals that influence a person's behaviour are likely to change (even if her values remain the same). The current concerns and tasks of a person recovering from ABI are to make sense of what has happened and to get fit and well. She may thus lose interest in some things that were previously important to her, including personal relationships. People with ABI are often described as egocentric, if not frankly selfish. As noted in Chapter 2, this may be a direct result of frontal lobe injury. But it is more often a sign of goals that have become much more tightly focused. These people are faced with a confusing and frightening situation, but have reduced cognitive resources with which to manage it. Just thinking about how to get through the day and then doing it may use all these resources. There is thus nothing left over to give to other people.

Sometimes ABI can be the occasion for a reordering of personal priorities, and this process can be experienced as positive and meaningful (Collicutt McGrath and Linley 2006). Changes in priorities (and occasionally even changes in values) may occur in response to the experience of brain injury. This is one reason that advance directives must be treated with caution. In addition, the situation anticipated in advance directives may not match the actual situation as it is experienced. (Advance directives are now covered by the Mental Capacity Act 2005.)

3.3.4 Social place

Part of being who we are is the way we assume and move between certain roles, such as being a parent, lover, friend, employee, student, carer, sportsperson, and so on. Roles give us a place or position in society and describe our relationships with others. In terms of the WHO-ICF model they define the degree and type of our participation. Some roles, such as 'medical practitioner', 'priest', 'adoptive parent' are conferred formally by specially designated groups within society. But all roles are the product of social construction, and to this extent so are our individual identities:

> The ways which we participate with this [social and cultural] matrix and construct identities that take up positions within this matrix, are through policy, contract, and institution ... Human identity is thus ... a historical contingency constituted in part by policies articulated by the social group, rather than as an underlying cognitive nature of the individual ... (Clocksin 1998, p. 118).

People with ABI relinquish many of their previous roles through a combination of activity limitation, broken relationships, and the attitudes of society (Olver 1996; Webster *et al.* 1999; Teasell *et al.* 2000). A person who is no longer 'husband', 'employee', 'householder', 'pub quiz champion' is in a very profound sense no longer his old self.

In addition, society is all too ready to confer new, undifferentiated, and lowly roles such as 'patient', 'service user', 'client', or 'disabled person' upon him. These lowly roles are often characterized by a blurring of psychological boundaries and a loss of psychological privacy. Sensitive personal and social information that under normal circumstances would be held privately or kept within the family circle, is made accessible to the teams who care for these people. This compounds the loss of physical privacy and the blurring of the body boundaries described on p. 42.

3.3.5 Personal narratives

Personal identity is not a static, but a dynamic developing phenomenon. We make sense of who we are as much by reflecting on our past and planning our future as we do by responding to our present situation (Ricoeur 1988). For this reason memory plays an enormously important role in forming both the identity of individuals and groups. We know about our habitual behaviours, past roles, and relationships through our autobiographical memory, and one interpretative framework used by autobiographical memory involves the goals and values that also influence our future behaviour. Our sense of who we are is dependent on the construction of a set of reasonably coherent narratives based on past events (McAdams 1990, 1993). These are punctuated by 'self-defining memories' (Singer and Salovey 1993), for instance failing the 11+, discovering Jane Austen, visiting the land of one's birth, being presented to the Queen. The degree of coherence and the number of narratives probably varies between individuals. Events may be linked into coherent wholes through their relationship to enduring personal concerns and intentions (Dennett 2004). Memory and intention are also intimately related to our enduring values, opinions, allegiances, and commitments.

A loss of autobiographical memory as part of retrograde amnesia removes large portions of personal history and can thus devastate narratives about the self. Older adults may retain memories from the distant past, but these may be subjectively disconnected from present experience. Young adults with retrograde amnesia may lose much of what contributed to their sense of self, and as a result may experience profound perplexity about their identity (McGrath 1998).

Anterograde amnesia can also interfere with personal narratives by interrupting their construction, so that they lose continuity, while executive impairment may result in a loss of coherence, as already noted. Because narratives are largely (though not exclusively) verbal, language impairment also interferes with their construction (Moss *et al.* 2004). In the words of one patient with language impairment describing his daily existence:

> There are programmes but there is no project. There is no connection with a wider sense of purpose in my life.

Nevertheless, it is unusual for people with ABI to complain of interruptions or distortions to the moment by moment subjective stream of consciousness (other than during the early stages or as a result of *petit mal* seizures). In contrast to people with severe mental health problems such as schizophrenia, they retain some psychological sense of continuity and integrity (Collicutt McGrath and Linley 2006). Thus, on the whole, even when people with ABI say 'I have become a different person' they still retain a sense of 'I'. That is they are experiencing themselves as the same person with profoundly *different characteristics* (see also Ellis-Hill *et al.* 2000). One reason that those around them may experience a *different person* is because this sense of 'I' is not accessible to them.

3.4 **Implications for rehabilitation**

We have seen that brain injury has the capacity to remove human personal characteristics; to make a person less individual, distinctive, and autonomous; and to make a person profoundly different from the way she was before.

Therefore good practice in the healthcare of people with ABI begins with affirming their humanity and involves supporting their individuality and autonomy. Good ABI rehabilitation practice builds on this, and is devoted to their personal reconstruction.

Reconstruction requires knowledge of the past, in this case knowledge of the sort of person the patient was before his injury. Yet we are all people-in-becoming, and future possibilities endow present experience with a unified meaning. So our knowledge must extend to the patient's previous aspirations for the future, his personal strivings. We are aiming for him to be in a position to resume his life's journey, not to remain static, and not to start a new journey in a totally different direction. Yet we are faced with a situation that is profoundly changed, and with a good deal of uncertainty. Rehabilitation is therefore a deeply creative process that takes place in the context of great challenges. It involves forging links between the patient's past and his future because these links have been broken by brain injury. While all this is happening the present must also be made tolerable.

Thus, intrinsic to the rehabilitation process is the establishment and maintenance of hope. Rehabilitation programmes can often be lacking in this respect, with their emphasis on drawing the patient's newly acquired limitations to his attention and instilling a sense of realism, acceptance, or 'insight'. Yet our hopes for the future include the fantastic alongside the realistic—that we will be thin, get that dream job, meet a wonderful man, win the lottery, and so on. Unrealistic hopes can help get us up in the morning, keep us going, and give us pleasure and self-respect. People with ABI should be allowed to hold on to some of these dreams as they start to come to terms with reality (Elliott and Kurylo 2000). And reality itself can be invested with hope and hence with meaning. The basic philosophy underpinning rehabilitation is that ABI is not the end for the patient, that his life is worth living, that his life can get better. Otherwise it is a pointless exercise. Personal values and goals may need to be adjusted and reframed, but not necessarily abandoned.

The aim of rehabilitation is therefore to support the person with ABI in establishing a new sense of identity continuous with, but not stuck in, the past (McGrath 2004), while managing the medical complications, pain, and emotional distress that arise during the process. The aspects of personal identity reviewed in this chapter suggest that in practical terms this will involve:

- sensitivity to and respect for the patient's physical and psychological boundaries
- taking seriously issues related to her personal appearance
- treating her impairments
- optimizing her agency and liberty

- training her in meaningful activities
- supporting her in the resumption of valued roles and relationships
- helping her to integrate the experience into a meaningful personal narrative
- managing any associated physical and psychological conditions.

These are simply the characteristics of good person-centred[3] rehabilitation practice. In this chapter I have argued that person-centred rehabilitation is the approach of choice because of the nature of ABI. To quote two researchers in this area, '... disruption to a person's core sense of self [is] almost the *sine qua non* of brain injury ...' (Jackson and Manchester 2001).

Person-centred brain injury rehabilitation entails collaborative interdisciplinary team work (McGrath and Davis 1992; McGrath *et al.* 1995; Wade 1999; Collicutt McGrath 2007a). This is simply because few if any of the rehabilitation activities enumerated above are the province of one discipline. In addition, despite the rhetoric of some professions, no single discipline can claim expertise in all areas. The expertise of professionals tends to be defined in terms of the treatment of specific impairments or the training of specific activities—the bits and pieces of people—not the rehabilitation of the whole person. When working well, the interdisciplinary team facilitates the integration of the person who has been fragmented by brain injury.

However, person-centred interdisciplinary practice needs to be set in the broader context of the motivation behind practitioners' desire to do the right thing. Practitioners of goodwill want to act in the best interests of their patients and others who are involved, to make the situation better for them. In this they are driven by moral values, to which we now turn.

Suggestions for further reading

The references below take up some of the themes of this chapter including issues of personal freedom, critiques of mind–body dualism, social construction of the self, human strivings towards goals and a sense of self, the role of memory in constructing a personal narrative. Where appropriate, short sections of special interest have been indicated.

Bennett M and Hacker P (2003). *Philosophical foundations of neuroscience*, pp. 111–114, 231–235. Blackwell, Oxford.

Burkitt I (1992). *Social selves: theories of the social formation of personality*. Sage, London.

---

[3] Person-centred practice is at the basis of much British public health policy and indeed is the first 'Quality Requirement' of the National Service Framework for long-term (neurological) conditions (2005), which includes ABI within its remit.

Emmons R (1999). *The psychology of ultimate concerns*, pp. 15–42. Guilford, New York.

Franks, A (1995). *The wounded storyteller*, pp. 97–114. University of Chicago Press, Chicago, IL.

Lapper A (2005). *My life in my hands*. Simon and Schuster, New York.

Mackay DM (1991). *Behind the eye*, pp. 190–213. Blackwell, Oxford.

Schachter D (1996). *Searching for memory: the brain, the mind, and the past*, pp. 72–97. Basic Books, New York.

Singer JA and Salovey P (1993). *The remembered self: emotion and memory in personality*, pp. 9–81. The Free Press, New York.

References

Bennett M and Hacker P (2003). *Philosophical foundations of neuroscience*. Blackwell, Oxford.

Carver C and Scheier M (1990). Origins and function of positive and negative affect: a control process view. *Psychological Review* **97**, 19–36.

Clocksin W (1998). Artificial intelligence and human identity. In J Cornwell, ed. *Consciousness and human identity*, pp. 101–121. Oxford University Press, Oxford.

Collicutt McGrath J (2007a). Post acute rehabilitation following traumatic brain injury. In A Tyerman and N King, eds. *Psychological approaches to rehabilitation after traumatic brain injury*. Blackwell, Oxford (in press).

Collicutt McGrath J (2007b). Recovery and rehabilitation from brain injury. In S Joseph and PA Linley, eds. *Trauma, recovery and growth: positive psychological perspectives on posttraumatic stress*. Wiley, New York (in press).

Collicutt McGrath J and Linley PA (2006). Post-traumatic growth in acquired brain injury: a preliminary small scale study. *Brain Injury* **20**, 767–773.

Dennett D (2004). *Consciousness explained*. Penguin, Harmondsworth.

Department of Health (2005). *The National Service Framework for long-term conditions*. Department of Health, London.

Dewey J (1922/2002). *Human nature and conduct*. Dover, Mineola NY.

Douglas M (1966). *Purity and danger*. Routledge and Kegan Paul, London.

Elliott T and Kurylo (2000). Hope over acquired disability: lessons of a young woman's triumph. In C Snyder, ed. *Handbook of hope: theory, measures, and application*, pp. 373–386. Academic Press, San Diego CA.

Ellis-Hill C, Payne S and Ward (2000). Self-body split: issues of identity in physical recovery following a stroke. *Disability and Rehabilitation* **22**, 725–733.

Emmons R (1999). *The psychology of ultimate concerns*. Guilford, New York.

Geertz C (1984). 'From the native's point of view': On the nature of anthropological understanding. In R Schweder and R Levine , eds. *Culture theory: essays on mind, self, and emotion*, pp. 123–136. Cambridge University Press, Cambridge.

Ginsburg C (1999). Body-image, movement and consciousness: examples from a somatic practice in the Feldenkrais Method. *Journal of Consciousness Studies* **6**, 79–91.

Gurevitch Z (1989). The power of not understanding: the meeting of conflicting identities. *Journal of Applied Behavioral Science* **25**, 161–173.

Gurevitch Z (1990). The embrace: on the element of non-distance in human relations. *Sociological Quarterly* **31**, 187–201.

Happe F, Bronwell H and Winner E (1999). Acquired 'theory of mind' impairments following stroke. *Cognition* **70**, 211–240.

Hurley S (1998). *Consciousness in action.* Harvard University Press, Cambridge MA.

Jackson H and Manchester D (2001). Towards the development of brain injury specialists. *Neurorehabilitation* **16**, 27–40.

Langdon R (2003). Theory of mind and social dysfunction: psychological solipsism versus autistic asociality. In B Repacholi and V Slaughter, eds. *Individual differences in theory of mind*, pp. 241–269. Psychology Press, New York.

McAdams D (1990). Unity and purpose in human lives: the emergence of identity as the life story. In A Rabin, R Zucker, R Emmons and S Franck, eds. *Studying persons and their lives*, pp. 148–200. Springer, New York.

McAdams D (1993). *The stories we live by: personal myths and the making of the self.* Morrow, New York.

McGrath J (1998). *Fear following brain injury.* PhD thesis, Oxford Brookes University.

McGrath J (2004). Beyond restoration to transformation: positive outcomes in the rehabilitation of acquired brain injury. *Clinical Rehabilitation* **18**, 767–775.

McGrath J and Adams L (1999). Patient-centred goal planning: A systemic psychological therapy? *Topics in Stroke Rehabilitation* **6**, 43–50.

McGrath J and Davis A (1992). Rehabilitation: Where are we going and how do we get there? *Clinical Rehabilitation* **6**, 255–235.

McGrath J, Marks J and Davis A (1995). Towards interdisciplinary rehabilitation: further developments at Rivermead Rehabilitation Centre. *Clinical Rehabilitation* **9**, 320–326.

Moore P (2003). *Being me: What it means to be human.* John Wiley, Chichester.

Moss B, Parr S, Byng S and Petheram B (2004). 'Pick me up and not a down down, up up': How are the identities of people with aphasia represented in aphasia, stroke and disability websites? *Disability and Society* **19**, 753–768.

Norenzayan A and Heine S (2005). Psychological universals: What are they and how can we know? *Psychological Bulletin* **131**, 763–784.

Oddy M (1995). He's no longer the same person: How families adjust to personality change after head injury. In N Chamberlain, ed. *Traumatic brain injury rehabilitation*, pp. 167–180. Chapman and Hall, London.

Olver J (1996). Outcome following traumatic brain injury: a comparison between two and five years after injury. *Brain Injury* **10**, 841–848.

Prigatano G (1991). Disordered mind, wounded soul: the emerging role of psychotherapy in rehabilitation after brain injury. *Journal of Head Trauma Rehabilitation* **6**, 1–10.

Rafferty J (2003). *Champion of deaf people.* BMJ Career Focus (on line) 327, available from http://www.Careerfocus.bmjjournals.com/vo1327/issue7428/s189 [accessed 17.7.06].

Ricoeur P (1988). *Time and narrative*, Volume III. University of Chicago Press, Chicago, IL.

Sheldon K and Kasser T (1995). Coherence and congruence: two aspects of personality integration. *Journal of Personality and Social Psychology* **68**, 531–543.

Simpson G, Blaszczynski A and Hodgkinson, A (1999). Sex offending as a psychosocial sequela of traumatic brain injury. *Journal of Head Trauma Rehabilitation* **14**, 567–580.

Singer JA and Salovey P (1993). *The remembered self: emotion and memory in personality.* The Free Press, New York.

Skinner J (2000). My brain works ... my legs don't! Let's take the 'dis' out of disabilities. *Society for Technical Communication, Special Needs Committee Proceedings.* Available from http://www.stc.org/48thConf/postconf/MG2XSNCMission.pdf [accessed 17.7.06].

Teasell R, McRae M and Finestone H (2000). Social issues in the rehabilitation of younger stroke patients. *Archives of Physical medicine and Rehabilitation* **81**, 205–209.

Varela F, Thompson E and Rosch E (1991). *The embodied mind: cognition, science and human experience.* MIT Press, Cambridge MA.

Wade D (1999). Goal planning in stroke rehabilitation: Why? *Topics in Stroke Rehabilitation* **6**, 1–7.

Webster G, Daisley A and King N (1999). Relationship and family breakdown following traumatic brain injury: the role of the rehabilitation team. *Brain Injury* **13**, 593–603.

Witchalls B (2005). Interview with BBC Crimewatch. Available from http://www.bbc.co.uk/pressoffice/pressreleases/stories/2005/05_may/18/crime.shtml [accessed 17.7.06].

Chapter 4

Moral values:
What is the right thing?

In considering the effects of acquired brain injury (ABI), I have paid a good deal of attention to the characteristics of individual human persons. This is essential to any understanding of the nature of this group of health conditions, and to the healthcare of those affected by them. But there is another important reason for emphasizing the personal. The individual person is at the centre of many (though not all) conceptions of morality.

Morality concerns values—beliefs about what is good. This notion of 'good' can be very broad. In English it essentially refers to things being as they should, or as they were meant to be, an idea of great relevance to healthcare. *Kalos*, the ancient Greek word usually translated 'good', incorporates this notion of propriety, but also extends to include truth and beauty. It implies an understanding that morality concerns aesthetics as much as ethics. On this understanding moral actions are beautiful as well as right.

It is actually quite hard to separate the beautiful and pleasing that come through aesthetic creative practices from the right and true that come through ethical practices. Living the good life involves both, and they are intimately connected. This resonates with my assertion in Chapter 1 that ethical practice is not distinct from technical practice but is a special case of it, and that professional life is not distinct from personal life but is a special domain within it. (So while it makes sense to speak of work–leisure or work–home balance it does not make sense to speak of work-life balance. Work is part of life (Baumeister 1987).)

Like the good life, good rehabilitation incorporates practices that are at the same time both aesthetic and ethical. This is why some of the ethical principles that will emerge from moral arguments in this chapter look very like some of the practices of creative person-centred rehabilitation commended in Chapter 3.

Moral actions are actions that are congruent with the moral values of the actor; however, there is a big jump from holding a moral value to knowing how to apply it in a particular situation, and a big jump from knowing how to apply it and actually going ahead and doing just that (see for instance, Bernard *et al.* 1987). This is where ethics comes in. Ethics is the systematic study of moral values and their translations into standards and rules of personal and cultural practices. These are sometimes formally codified as laws, and sometimes gathered together more informally as part of the wisdom tradition of a culture, often in the form of proverbs or poems such as Kipling's 'If'. Cognitive therapists (Barnard and Teasdale 1993; Padesky and Greenberger 1995) have also drawn to our attention the importance of 'underlying assumptions' in the lives of individuals. These often barely articulated beliefs and rules (of the sort 'It's dangerous to trust strangers', 'I should try and put the needs of others first') are used by us all as a rough guide to everyday living, as part of a personal ethical system.

In this chapter I will discuss some aspects of moral theory and, on the basis of this discussion, generate some broad principles for ethical practice in the context of brain injury rehabilitation. Some of these practice principles may appear to conflict with each other. In Chapter 5 they will be developed further into specific guidelines, and potential conflicts will be explored.

Any approach to morality and ethics will be from a particular perspective. The approach I have taken is influenced by a number of different accounts of morality, in particular Judaeo-Christian, Kantian, and postmodern analyses. It also uses narrative as a way into understanding morality. Another author might have placed the emphasis elsewhere, perhaps on utilitarian theories and the tight methodology of deductive argument. My choice arises from my personal morality, is a response to the particular moral challenges that are posed by ABI, and bears in mind the need to communicate a highly complex and often controversial area with clarity and at least some coherence. It aims to show how acceptance of a particular approach to morality can be translated into principles and guidelines that make a practical difference to the way in which rehabilitation is delivered. That is, it aims to demonstrate the moral basis of certain clinical practices.

If morality concerns the good, then there is really only one moral principle. This is to do good to other persons—the principle of beneficence. The other side of the 'doing good' coin is not doing harm. This is the principle of non-maleficence.

4.1 **Non-maleficence**

The principle of non-maleficence is the least demanding moral principle. It is expressed frequently in statements like, 'It doesn't matter what you do so long as you don't harm anyone else.' This principle is common to most major religions and philosophies, often stated in terms of a 'golden rule'. A very early version of this, dating from 500 BCE is the Confucian saying 'Do not do to others what you would not like yourself.' (Analects 12:2). In defining harm to others as something that would be harmful to me, the golden rule introduces the important idea that other people are essentially like me.

In addition to inflicting harm, maleficent behaviour is usually understood to include negligence—that is imposing risk of harm. All members of society are expected to behave towards the people they come across in the course of their daily life with non-maleficence. They may also have an obligation of non-maleficence to people they have never met, but who might reasonably be thought to come within their sphere of responsibility.

The principle of non-maleficence clearly applies to healthcare professionals in their contact with their patients. They are under an obligation not to inflict harm and not to expose to risk of harm. *Primum non nocere* ('first do no harm') is a basic principle of medical practice dating back to the Roman physician Galen.

Practice principle 2. Don't make things worse

Very rarely, as in the infamous case of Dr Harold Shipman, health professionals set out to harm their patients. Their behaviour is unambiguously immoral and illegal, and presents few if any ethical dilemmas. More usually harm is inflicted unintentionally as a result of error, or in pursuit of a higher level goal (for instance, the amputation of a limb in order to save a patient's life). Ethical questions may sometimes be raised by these situations.

In other cases there is disagreement about what constitutes harm. This issue is highlighted by the controversy surrounding the removal of nasogastric or gastrostomy tubes providing food and water to patients in persisting minimal awareness states. On one analysis, while the insertion of a tube and the introduction of nutrients directly into the alimentary canal can take place without the permission of the patient in an emergency, once the acute emergency is past its continuing use constitutes involuntary treatment, and is tantamount to physical assault. It contravenes the principle of non-maleficence because it inflicts harm through invading the patient's body, and is futile in that it offers nothing that can improve the patient's situation. It is a type of assault. On an alternative analysis, withdrawal of the nutrients necessary to keep the patient alive, ceasing to provide basic care, contravenes the principle of non-maleficence because it imposes a 100% risk of death from starvation. It is a type of neglect (Finnis 1993). This example shows that defining harm and welfare in any given situation is not always simple, and the use of charged terms such as 'futile', 'assault', 'care', and 'starvation' can confuse things further.

4.2 **Beneficence**

The principle of beneficence, actively doing good through the promotion of welfare and the prevention and removal of harm, finds one expression in the positive version of the golden rule, 'In everything do to others as you would have them do to you' (Matthew 7.12a). This is clearly a more exacting standard than its non maleficent cousin. This particular form of words is not found outside the Christian tradition, though the notion of loving one's neighbour as oneself is more widespread.

The application of the principle of beneficence is generally more restricted than the principle of non-maleficence. In most societies it is understood to apply to only certain types of relationships. This may be for simple practical reasons. Doing good generally takes more time, energy, and resources, than not doing harm. Some priorities need to be established and some limits set.

For instance, on this understanding, a food production company has an obligation to promote the interests of its shareholders. It does not have an obligation to promote the interests of the people who buy and eat its products. But it does have an obligation not to cause them harm by selling them cheap contaminated products to increase its profits.

Or a father has an obligation to promote the welfare of his children by providing them with food. He does not have an obligation to promote the welfare of other children in his neighbourhood. But he does have an obligation not to cause these other children harm by taking food away from them to feed his own children.

Again, a nurse has an obligation to promote the welfare of patients on her unit by carrying out an agreed plan of care. She does not have an obligation to promote the welfare of patients on other units in her hospital. But she does have an obligation not to cause harm to patients on other units, for instance by encouraging one of her patients to visit a friend in another unit if he has an easily transmissible condition such as methicillin-resistant *Staphylococcus aureus* (MRSA).

In each of these instances there is an obligation of beneficence to a small group and an obligation of non-maleficence to a larger group. This type of restriction in the obligation of beneficence is sometimes overridden, often in emergencies where a danger to life is involved. For instance, if there is a fire in the hospital the nurse may be required to promote the welfare of all patients by taking part in a general evacuation.

On the face of it all this seems reasonable, yet it invites two very significant questions. The first question is 'What does it actually mean to do good?' (If we assume that harm is the opposite of good, an answer to this question will also illuminate the principle of non-maleficence.) The second question is 'With whom am I in the special sort of relationship that requires me to do good?'

In exploring these two questions I will use a story. Stories are helpful because they are vivid, engaging, personal, and have coherent narrative structure. This particular story is ancient, has been extremely influential in Western culture—even cited in English negligence law (Donoghue v Stevenson 1932), and concerns the healthcare of a person who almost certainly sustained a head injury as the result of an assault.

> '… A man was going down from Jerusalem to Jericho, and fell into the hands of robbers, who stripped him, beat him, and went away, leaving him half dead. Now by chance a priest was going down that road; and when he saw him, he passed by on the other side. So likewise a Levite, when he came to the place and saw him, passed by on the other side. But a Samaritan while travelling came near him; and when he saw him, he was moved with pity. He went to him and bandaged his wounds, having poured oil and wine on them. Then he put him on his own animal, brought him to an inn, and took care of him. The next day he took out two denarii, gave them to the innkeeper, and said, 'Take care of him; and when I come back, I will repay you whatever more you spend.' Which of these three, do you think, was a neighbour to the man who fell into the hands of the robbers?' [The lawyer] said, 'The one who showed him mercy.' Jesus said to him, 'Go and do likewise.'
>
> Luke 10. 30–37 (New Standard Revised Version)

4.2.1 What is good?

In the gospel of Luke this story is presented in the context of a discussion that is essentially about how to live a good life. A Jewish lawyer reflects on the teaching from the ancient Hebrew book of Leviticus (Leviticus 19.18) that one is required to love one's neighbour as oneself—a moral value that forms the basis of much of the ethical system that is the Jewish law. This form of the positive golden rule is crucially stated in terms of an *attitude* (an enduring disposition), in this case 'love', rather than in terms of emotion or behaviour.

Like the other two versions of the golden rule we considered earlier, this one rests on an assumption that the individual towards whom my beneficence is directed is essentially like me. I know how I would like to be treated. I know how I would not like to be treated. I look out for my own best interests—that is I love myself. To be beneficent is to think and act as if the recipient of my beneficence were actually me.

This requires a mental rotation. Instead of seeing the other as somebody to whom my actions are directed, I have to turn myself around and inhabit her perspective as someone who is herself directing action. This is perhaps the most important difference between seeing somebody as an object and seeing her as a person. Some philosophers have argued that it is the essential difference. To recognize the agency and capacity of the other for autonomy is to see her as a person like me. It is the basis of beneficence. The converse attitude is depicted by the pejorative phrase 'do-gooder'. This is used to refer to someone who may behave with kindness and generosity but treats others as objects on which this kindness and generosity are bestowed, as pawns in his own pseudo-beneficent agenda, as means to his own ends rather than as ends in themselves.

The golden rule has emerged in many different societies essentially on the basis of intuition. The philosopher Immanuel Kant (1724–1804) provides a systematic (and difficult) argument for it that rests on the supremacy of human reason. Kant argues that morality both makes us aware that we can be free, and has the potential to make us free, because it confronts us with genuine choices. But, in an anticipation of the findings of twentieth century psychologists (see for example Wilson and Dunn 2003), he observes that the choices we make are all too often determined by our own assumptions, desires, and agendas. These he views as part of our non-rational nature, arising from our 'lower passions', which include our emotions. If we are to act in a truly moral way, to make really autonomous choices, we need somehow to transcend these desires and agendas and to be dispassionate. Kant argues that it is only possible to do this and to arrive at a truly objective view of right action if we ignore the intended consequences of our actions and concentrate on the actions in themselves. This is because intended consequences often relate to our agendas, but actions considered on their own cannot. That is, if we are to be truly moral we should think of actions as ends in themselves and not as means to ends. Moral principles should therefore be stated in terms of actions or attitudes only, and not in terms of their intended consequences or the specific circumstance in which they arise. The technical term for this type of moral principle is 'categorical imperative'. For example, 'Always tell the truth' is a type of categorical imperative; 'Tell the truth if it is to your advantage' is not. According to Kant there are a number of fundamental rules or formulae on which categorical imperatives should be based. The two most important are presented below.

The first formula 'Of Universal Law' states that if a moral principle is to be 'objective' or disinterested it should apply to me just as much as to everyone else, and should therefore relate to what any rational being would view as right action. '... act only in accordance with that maxim through which you at the same time can will that it become a universal law.' (Groundwork 4: 421, cf. 4; 402). This should lead me, for instance, to hold to a principle of never stealing because although stealing might meet my need for personal gain, no rational being would want to live in world where others could freely steal from her (a rationalist version of the golden rule).

But there is more. I am only a truly free moral agent through embracing an autonomous choice to behave according to this kind of rational golden rule.

I do this because I want to be free. Therefore, by the golden rule, I must want others to be free. I am required to respect their agency and capacity for autonomous and distinctive choice; I must not treat them as objects. This second formula 'Of Humanity as an End in Itself' states 'So act that you use humanity—as much in your own person as in the person of every other—always at the same time as an end and never merely as a means.' (Groundwork 4: 429, cf. 4: 436). Note Kant's emphasis that this attitude should be applied to me as much as to other people. It is a way of caring for myself. By respecting the distinctive identity and freedom of all people I also achieve my own distinctive identity and freedom.

This is the ancient command to love one's neighbour seen from the rationalist and idealist perspective of the eighteenth century Age of Enlightenment. It emphasizes an attitude to the other that recognizes and respects, and may go so far as to promote, her autonomy. It has been highly influential and has much to commend it. In Chapter 3 I laboured the point that people with ABI are in 'autonomy deficit' because of restrictions arising from impairment and context. Kant's approach is thus particularly applicable to thinking about what beneficence might mean in the context of ABI (Rosenthal and Lourie 1996). It at least seems like a reasonable place to start.

> *Practice principle 3.* Promote the agency, distinctive identity, and freedom of the patient.

4.2.2 Who is my neighbour?

To return to the story of the Good Samaritan, the lawyer who is reflecting on the requirement to love one's neighbour asks Jesus the obvious question that arises from it, 'Who is my neighbour?' The text at this point remarks that his motive in doing this is to 'justify himself'. That is he is looking to set some limits on the principle of beneficence.

The story is told in response to this theoretical question about morality, but it is framed in the rather different terms of practical action and human emotion. This rich and nuanced narrative depicts in some detail what 'doing good' might actually look like. The picture it paints has a high degree of simple face validity. Thus we are told that the lawyer immediately recognizes the moral action of the Samaritan for what it is.

Yet the story is radical and subversive. Its most distinctive feature is that the act of beneficence is carried out by someone who does not have a recognized duty of care for its recipient. It is assumed that the victim of the assault is a Jew. The person who helps him is ethnically and religiously different.

There are no national or family ties of obligation. Indeed there was a well-attested and longstanding tradition of mutual animosity between Jews and Samaritans. Nevertheless the Samaritan in this story acts towards this stranger as if a duty of care is required. Furthermore, because the victim has lost all his money and is probably unconscious the Samaritan cannot expect payment or even thanks from him. There is no opportunity for reciprocity. The Samaritan in many ways meets the requirements of Kant's account of morality. His actions are not driven by natural affection for his own kind, or suspicion of difference, or hope of reward. They are good actions directed at the victim as an end in himself.

The Greek word that is translated 'neighbour' in this story can also mean 'fellow human being'. In modern English we have the same double meaning for the word 'close'—which can mean either geographical proximity or emotional/familial intimacy. Note how the story emphasizes that the Samaritan 'came near' and 'went to' the injured Jew. The challenge to the hearer is to expand his horizons with regard to who is close to him, not only as a fellow human being (Practice principle 1 from Chapter 3 flows directly from this attitude) but as someone whose welfare is his concern.

The story is critical of an approach to beneficence that limits its application too strictly. It suggests, in some sense, that the food company of our earlier example may actually have an obligation to promote the welfare of its customers, the father may have an obligation to promote the welfare of other children on his street, and the nurse may have an obligation to promote the welfare of patients in other units. In the case of ABI, it invites practitioners to reflect on the nature of their obligation to carers, family, and friends, to other professionals on the team, to patients on the unit who are not their direct responsibility, and on their contribution to situations that seem to stray outside the boundaries of their professional remit.

Practice principle 4. Think outside the box: your moral responsibility may extend further than you thought

A crucial part of the description of beneficence in this story is the detail that the Samaritan was 'moved with pity'—he experienced compassion. In this respect he departs dramatically from Kant's account of morality. Instead of acting according to an exclusively rational principle the Samaritan does what *feels* right. He is emotionally moved, and this tells us that he has indeed ceased to see the victim as distant and different from himself and instead sees him as essentially close and similar. He has transcended prejudice by empathic emotion—what some philosophers call the 'moral impulse'—rather than by the application of dispassionate reason (Vetlesen 1993).

Postmodern philosophers, while welcoming Kant's vision of a morality that is purged of self-interest, have criticized his assertion that reason uncontaminated by emotion is the way to achieve it. In this respect they are more in tune with the Samaritan in this story. They agree with Kant that the essence of morality is to treat the other as a person, free from my own agenda, and expecting nothing in return. But they point out that morality refers to *relationships* between real people who feel as well as think.

> ... to delegitimize or 'bracket away' moral impulses and emotions, and then to try to reconstruct the edifice of ethics out of arguments carefully cleansed of emotional undertones and set free from all bonds with unprocessed human intimacy, is equivalent ... to saying that if we could get the walls out of the way we would better see what supports the ceiling. [Emotion] is the primal and primary 'brute fact' of moral impulse, moral responsibility, moral intimacy that supplies the stuff from which the morality of human cohabitation is made.
>
> Bauman (1993 p. 35)

If this analysis is correct, it implies that much of what we traditionally take to be 'professional' behaviour—keeping emotionally distant, adopting a position of clinical detachment, not allowing emotion to cloud our judgement, not expressing emotion in the professional setting—lacks moral characteristics. It is perhaps amoral. It is certainly unnatural. If health professionals do not express emotion during formal clinical activities, they will readily do so in more informal settings. This is presumably why clinical teams feel the need to 'de-brief' after difficult meetings or procedures; why individuals may seek each other out to express emotions such as frustration, indignation, and sorrow, and to reflect on what they are doing; and why through this natural, informal, emotional, and moral process relationships between team members are often strengthened. It is impossible and also undesirable to keep emotion out of the picture.

Practice principle 5. Welcome and make proper use of empathic and other emotion as a basis for moral action

Practice principle 6. Acknowledge the emotional experience of the patient and address her emotional needs

It is possible to design a standard of practice that states that practitioners will treat other people as fellow human beings, but human emotions are beyond the control of such legislation. They thus present a management challenge when they arise in professional situations. It should also be added that once emotion and empathy are acknowledged to be part of the picture, and morality is seen to involve feeling, we start to see that it is costly. The story of the Good Samaritan mentions the monetary cost explicitly; however, empathic action also involves time, effort, and a degree of emotional pain.

There is much potential for empathy in brain injury rehabilitation, and it can often be the cause of problems. As we have already noted, ABI affects previously fit and healthy individuals. It is no respecter of social class, education, or age. Thus, while the patient with ABI is in so many respects deeply unlike those caring for her, the same patient may *previously* have been very like some of them. This is one reason that it can be such a shock to see photographs of a patient before her injury. An immediate sense of the person she used to be is communicated. This can make us sad, as we come to understand what has been lost. It can make us perplexed as we ponder the connection between the patient we think we know and the person in the photograph. But it can also make us anxious, as we realize first that she is 'like me', and then that 'this could happen to me.'

This is deeply threatening. To work every day with people who have been struck down by illness and injury with devastating results, and yet to survive psychologically requires us to distance ourselves from this threat, so that we can preserve core assumptions that the world is safe, benevolent, or meaningful (Janoff-Bulman 1992). Being courteous but maintaining distance, treating bits and pieces of people (and thereby exacerbating the fragmentation already wrought by brain injury), focusing on an arm or a leg rather than the whole person, emphasizing the professional–patient rather than the person–person nature of the relationship, all protect us from empathy and allow us to do a professional job.

Perhaps a rationalist approach to morality is better after all? Empathy is painful. It may get in the way of our ability to function efficiently. It may also mislead us into bad decisions. One of the cases discussed during the fictional admissions meeting in Chapter 1 was that of a university student whose cause was taken up by a junior doctor. The young man reminded her of her own brother. She perceived his family as like her own family. His situation touched her deeply— it called up a moral impulse. But she had become so emotionally involved that instead of being merely disappointed that the team could not offer him immediate admission she was devastated. Her empathy was emotionally costly and, it seems, distorted her professional judgement. It was a kind of selective empathy. She had come to believe that this young man should take precedence over all other patients on the waiting list. But how could that be just?

4.2.3 **What about justice?**

We can only respond with empathy to people with whom we have had personal contact. What about the interests of those we have not seen or do not know? We are more likely to feel empathy towards people we perceive as like us. What about those we perceive as unlike us? We are more likely to respond with goodwill towards 'lovable' or attractive people. What about those who are 'unlovable' or unattractive? Empathy is a start but it is not sufficient to ensure fair practice. Utilitarian philosophers from John Stuart Mill onwards have rightly drawn attention to the need for a consistent assessment of the interests of *all*, and a transparent and impartial means of making decisions that affect them.

Practice principle 7. Take all interested parties into account

The question of justice arises when there is a conflict between the interests of an individual and the interests of others. Again, emotion has a part to play. However, rather than empathy, it is feelings of unease or frank indignation that can alert us to issues of injustice. Issues of justice become particularly relevant in cases where resources are limited. There is no doubt that brain injury rehabilitation can be extremely expensive. Whether privately or publicly funded, resources are always limited. Therefore, the idealistic aim of rehabilitation as described on p. 47 will always need to be worked out in a real situation in the light of the available resources.

Practice principle 8. Be realistic about available resources

What would the Samaritan have done if he had come across a group of people who had been attacked, all of whom needed help? He would presumably have had to set some priorities.

The problem comes in deciding how to set priorities. We will briefly consider three alternative methods of setting priorities in healthcare, all aimed at establishing distributive justice (fair provision of resources). The first method is to consider overall net gain—the greatest good for the greatest number. This method begins by asking who is most likely to benefit from input, or who could potentially put more back into society—for instance by resuming gainful employment—therefore benefiting other interested parties in addition to themselves, or who can afford to pay (from private funds or via proxy purchasing procedures)—thereby contributing to the healthcare service. In Chapter 1 both the doctor's assumption that the needs of a young adult should take priority over the needs of an older adult, and the group's discussion about the knock-on effects of admitting a heavily dependent patient to a mixed unit were influenced by this essentially utilitarian perspective.

In practice it may prove very difficult to implement a utilitarian approach to the distribution of rehabilitation resources for people with brain injury. This is for a number of reasons. First, while it is possible to construct statistical models of variables that predict outcome after brain injury (e.g. Fleming *et al.* 1999), the high degree of variability in this population means that predicting the outcome for any individual patient remains extremely difficult (Wade 1999). Again, neurological rehabilitation is a young and rapidly developing speciality, and its techniques are poorly standardized and only partially evaluated. The effectiveness of a proposed intervention with a specific individual in a local clinical setting is thus also very difficult to predict (Swiercinsky 2002). Finally, what constitutes a 'good outcome' is highly debatable. From a utilitarian perspective it is probably most easily and reliably defined in terms of how much a person costs the state, with the optimum outcome being financial self-sufficiency. However, this sort of definition would not be acceptable to many (Banja and Johnston 1994; Malec 1996), and in practical terms it is rarely achieved by people with severe ABI.

Another problem with the utilitarian method, specifically with respect to the needs of people with ABI, is that it is designed to maximize the interests of the majority. In most cases it is in a person's interests to comply with a utilitarian system because the odds are that what is in the interests of the whole group will also be in his interests. However, this may not hold true for minority groups. In healthcare, people with rare conditions or conditions of extreme severity and complexity may be penalized by a system that is geared to the average. At a national level specialist services for younger adults with the mix of problems arising from severe ABI have traditionally attracted less attention than services for the larger numbers of older adults with brain disease or younger adults with predominantly physical disabilities. On the other hand some people with ABI are in receipt of substantial settlements from insurance companies, and can thus make a useful financial contribution in the role of purchasers. These individuals are likely to benefit from systems based on utilitarian principles because what they may cost the state is offset by what they can pay. (However, see Macleod and Smith 2005 on the converse relative difficulty in accessing rehabilitation services for some deprived groups.)

A feature of the utilitarian method is that it treats people as means alone rather than ends in themselves, as small cogs in the large wheel of the general good. It is therefore inconsistent with the Kantian and postmodern approaches to morality that I have been commending earlier in this chapter.

For essentially pragmatic reasons individuals are appraised primarily in terms of their potential to contribute to society. It can be a short step from this to a method that views the ultimate value of individuals in these terms.

The second method for setting priorities that we shall consider does precisely this. It looks at individual cases in terms of merit or moral deservingness. From a utilitarian perspective it might be argued that it is inadvisable to waste expensive heart surgery on a heavy smoker who does not intend to quit, because the chances of adding significantly to the general good in terms of productive years of life are low in comparison with treating a non-smoker. A system based on merit might reach the same conclusion but for rather different reasons. The argument here would be that a heavy smoker who knew the risks associated with his habit has contributed to his own situation and is less *deserving* of treatment than a non-smoker. He is worth less in moral as well as practical terms (see Harris 1985). In Chapter 1 the question of the appropriateness of placing a street drinker on a waiting list for costly rehabilitation was presented as arising from a utilitarian perspective, but to some of those present it felt like a judgement on his intrinsic merit as a human being.

It is easy for arguments based on the general good to shade almost imperceptibly into arguments about the ultimate worth of persons. It is also easy for arguments about the worth of persons to move from the philosophical or theological discourses where they belong into more empirical discourses concerning notions such as 'quality of life', 'happiness', or 'satisfaction.' However, understandings of what 'quality of life' actually mean are so variable, and often vague, that it is arguably impossible to achieve reliable or meaningful measurement (see Murray and Acharya 1997; Brock 1998; Nord 1999; Addington-Hall and Kara 2001; Farside and Dunlop 2001; Carr *et al.* 2002 for a range of views). Happiness and life satisfaction are complex notions that are often difficult to capture and are not related in any simple way to variables that are more easily measured, such as wealth and physical health (Albrecht and Devilieger 1999; Guiton 2002). There is also an ethical problem. If we think we can operationalize the value of individuals in terms of measurable features such as life expectancy, degree of disability, happiness levels, sexual preference, race, or religion, we are flirting with the mind set that found its extreme expression in the twentieth century Third Reich.

We have seen that basing treatment and care priorities on potential overall gain in utility, or improvement in life quality, is practically difficult, especially in the area of brain injury rehabilitation. Utilitarian systems can all too easily and unwittingly become meritocracies. Meritocracies assign differential value to individuals and this is morally disquieting. If we wish to avoid the disadvantages of utilitarian systems or meritocracies we will choose the third alternative—'fair shares for all'—a method that is strictly egalitarian, which treats the claims of all as of equal value and responds accordingly. But what does it mean to respond accordingly? Does it mean providing equal access to, or speed of, or total amount of treatment, or all three? Does it mean equal treatment for all, or should treatment instead be in proportion to an individual's needs? People with ABI are highly variable and a 'one size fits all' approach to rehabilitation seems unlikely to be the fairest basis on which to allocate resources. But if individually tailored approaches are to be preferred, how should they be managed in order to be fair? In a context where resources are limited, the rationing imposed by a 'fair shares for all' system may mean that everybody receives an equally inadequate service (Doyal 1995; Butler 1999; Cookson and Dolan 2000; Daniels and Sabin 2002).

Formal schemes to help decide these sorts of questions can be set up at local or national level, and this is surely good practice. Transparency and uniformity of methods, clarity of definition, and measurable criteria are important features of such schemes, which aim at 'procedural justice'—ensuring that the *process* of resource allocation is both fair and seen to be fair. (Procedural justice feels attainable even if distributive justice remains elusive.) These schemes are usually based on an uneasy combination of utilitarianism and egalitarianism: 'the greatest good for the greatest number' and 'fair shares for all' both seem good principles but do not sit easily alongside each other.

At the local level a service that carries out formal triage to assess and set priorities, or has published standards of practice that address the cost-effectiveness of the treatment it offers, or has a systematic approach to the management of its waiting list(s) is practising procedural justice and aiming at distributive justice (for a more detailed discussion see Scott 1998). At the national level the British National Health Service (NHS) is served in this respect by the National Institute for Health and Clinical Effectiveness (NICE). This organization is explicitly driven by a moral agenda of distributive justice in the context of limited government departmental budgets. It is largely, though not exclusively, utilitarian in its approach, and takes some pains to safeguard itself against a slide into meritocratic values (NICE 2005). Good quality information about the effectiveness of treatments for specific health conditions is thus vital for its operation.

Despite their conceptual complexity and practical limitations, formal protocols, procedures, and standards have a big part to play in the establishment and maintenance of transparent and consistent practice. They also draw our attention to the moral issue of justice, and can help manage emotion and conflict, so that just decisions are more likely to occur.

Practice principle 9. Use, and if necessary develop, practice standards and protocols to temper emotion

Nevertheless, according to Kant, these sorts of systems have the capacity to stifle personal morality. This sounds mad. How can a system designed to promote the general good and/or safeguard the interests of individuals result in a reduction in moral action? Kant argues that this occurs through the elimination of our free autonomous choice (see also Bauman 1993, pp. 124–125). If we have a system and we do everything by the book we essentially pass the buck, and hence lose any sense of personal involvement in the making of moral decisions. This makes theoretical sense in light of what psychology tells us about the inverse relationship between extrinsic rewards and intrinsic motivation (Lepper *et al.* 1996). The empirical evidence also suggests that the presence of a code of conduct makes people no more likely to behave according to its standards unless it is enforced with rewards and sanctions (Matthews 1987; Ford and Richardson 1994), and that codes of conduct can actually have a detrimental effect on moral behaviour (Bandura *et al.* 1996). This seems to be because moral responsibility no longer rests with the individual practitioner but has been relocated in the system (Bandura 1999; Beauchamp and Childress 2001, p. 191).

Practice standards and protocols arise in response to moral problems, often concerning justice, but their routine implementation can lead to a losing sight of what they were all about in the first place. The sting in the tail of the story of the Good Samaritan is precisely this point. Two people 'pass by on the other side'. They make sure that they keep their distance from the person who is in need. But they do not do this out of malice or unconcern. They do it in order to comply with what were essentially professional practice demands. They take a utilitarian approach. In order to maintain the well-being of the nation priests and Levites were required to remain ritually clean. Coming close to a person who was dead and dying would have made them unclean and, in terms of their world view, would have compromised the greater good (Leviticus 21.1). The reluctance of this priest and Levite to violate their ethical code inhibits their freedom to make a moral choice. Yet this code itself arose originally from a genuine desire to do good.

Practice principle 10. Do not be enslaved to practice standards and protocols

What are we to conclude? It seems that it is unrealistic and undesirable to eliminate empathic emotion as a component of ethical practice. Yet this emotion has to be managed. We need systematic protocols and standards of practice. These are especially important when there are conflicts of interest and limited resources. Yet it is all too easy to hide behind these systems and to use them to avoid moral responsibility and genuine ethical practice.

In fact we need to be able to hold both the moral impulse and the ethical system together. They are useful counterpoints to each other. Each, in its own way 'helps us extricate ourselves from narrow egocentricity' (Watts 2004, p. 62). We need to realize that the moral impulse and the ethical system are in constant tension, accept that there will never be perfect resolution between them, and learn to live with the disquiet that this can cause. We need, as it were, to listen to our hearts *and* think with our heads (Haidt 2001). We also need to recognize that conflict in interdisciplinary teams may be a healthy working out of this tension rather than a sign of dysfunction (Jehn 1994, 1995).

4.2.2 The problem of paternalism

We can fairly safely assume that the man who was helped by the Samaritan would, if conscious, have consented to the treatment and care he received. But what if he had asked to be left alone to die? The problem of paternalism arises when what appears to be in the patient's best interests does not promote his agency, distinctive identity, and freedom.

Parents face this with their children all the time despite protests—limiting their intake of sweets, not letting them play with fire, putting them to bed early, and so on. There is an understanding that children are not in a position fully to appreciate the consequences of their actions. There is also an understanding that this is a temporary state of affairs, that children will gradually (or quite suddenly in some cultures) cease to require such restrictions. They will be deemed to have the capacity to make autonomous choices, even if these turn out to be bad choices.

In some respects people with ABI can seem rather like children. They may need help with washing and dressing. They may be wheeled around in a larger version of a push-chair. They may have to learn, or be taught by experts, to walk and talk, to ride a bicycle, to read and write. They may seem emotionally immature, indulging in 'tantrums' or weeping freely. Their behaviour can seem uncontrolled and 'naughty'. They may not have a full appreciation of their situation or the consequences of their intended action.

The 'brain injury = second childhood' model is in some ways appealing to the adult parents of people with ABI. It gives them a handle on the situation. They know the right way to behave towards children and, crucially, they can remember when the patient actually was a child for whom they were responsible. In some ways they can step back and enter a previous mode of being with that person. This option is not open to the patient's life partner. When Alison described her husband as a third child in Chapter 1, she was essentially saying that the marital relationship was over.

But of course adults with brain injury are not children. Children are on a developmental trajectory characterized by hope, celebrated at each birthday with the endowment of more freedom and a vision for the future. People with ABI are adults who once knew agency and liberty, have lost much of what they had, and whose future prospects of regaining them are uncertain. Further restricting their opportunities for autonomy is ethically questionable (Practice principle 3) and cannot be informed by a paternalistic model (Bauman 1993, pp. 120–121). Clearly restrictions may be necessary to protect the interests of other people (Practice principle 7). It would be unethical to encourage a patient with ABI to drive on the open road if it put others at risk. But restrictions invoked for the patient's 'own good' are a different matter.

Practice principle 11. Give greatest weight to the agency, distinctive identity, and freedom of the patient when considering what is in his or her interests.

People with ABI may find it difficult to make good choices because they may not fully appreciate their situation and the consequences of intended courses of action. This may be because of cognitive impairment or because the relevant information has not been shared with them. In addition they may have difficulty communicating their wishes clearly because of speech or language impairment. The onus is then on the practitioner to address these issues. This will be explored in some detail in Chapter 5. The decisions in question may relate to consenting to a course of treatment, getting married, spending money, participating in dangerous leisure activities and so on. Each should be treated on its own merits.

Practice principle 12. Assess and maximize the patient's competence/capacity to make specific decisions and communicate his or her wishes

However, this assessment may demonstrate that the patient lacks the competence/capacity to make an autonomous choice even under the most favourable circumstances. In these cases paternalistic action to protect her interests is probably justified, though (in line with Practice principle 3) the least autonomy-restrictive action should be chosen. Taking a paternalistic decision may be necessary but it can cause great distress.

> *Practice principle 13.* Acknowledge and manage distress caused by necessary paternalistic action

But what if the patient is in possession of the relevant information about her situation, seems to understand the consequences of a proposed course of action, and can communicate her wishes clearly, but the proposed course of action seems inadvisable? The answer to this question depends on the nature of the envisaged consequences. The argument for overriding her wishes is strongest if there is a very high risk of significant harm (death, severe physical injury, significant mental ill health). If the risk is low or the type of harm is less clear-cut (emotional exploitation or humiliation, loss of money or possessions, minor or moderate physical injury) the argument for paternalistic action is much less strong. Many people take inadvisable risks in the course of their everyday lives. They get into bad relationships, neglect or damage their health, or are profligate with money. They indulge in activities that might not accord with my understanding of what it is to live a good life—my moral values. Yet if we accept that ethical practice is about promoting individual freedom to choose, we must also accept that we cannot impose our values upon other people, including our patients.

> *Practice principle 14.* Do not impose your personal or professional values on the patient

It might be argued in response that health professionals have a particular duty of care for their patients, and this extends to preventing them from making bad choices. This duty of care does not extend to the general public. One way of elaborating and bolstering up this position is to argue that bad decision making is a defining feature of some types of brain injury. It is a symptom that needs to be managed and treated. By this account bad choices become components of syndromes or diseases. The most controversial yet powerful of these is 'dysexecutive syndrome'. (For a range of perspectives on 'dysexecutive syndrome' see Duncan *et al.* 1997; Baddeley 1998; Burgess *et al.* 1998; Parkin 1998; Chan 2001.) The medicalization of bad choices is dangerous and needs to be resisted. 'Healthcare of' can become 'power over'; clinical responsibility can become oppression (Bauman 1993, p. 91).

People who have problems in thinking because of executive or other cognitive impairment may indeed have a greater tendency to make choices that we would regard as imprudent. But each of these choices needs to examined and managed on its own merits, not from the starting point that the patient must be wrong because he has a particular type of cognitive impairment, or wrong just because he has ABI. Sometimes patients are right and professionals are wrong, sometimes there is a genuine difference of opinion (McGrath and King 2004, p. 347). Sometimes benefits may come from making what seems to be a bad choice, and appropriate care takes the form of thinking through the experience with the patient afterwards rather than protecting him from it in advance.

Practice principle 15. Clarify the nature and extent of your duty of care

There remains the difficult problem of whose autonomy we are upholding if the patient makes a bad choice that is totally out of character with his pre-injury values. Are we really doing him any favours by supporting his right to make this choice? A simple answer to this is that we are where we are. Nevertheless, as discussed on page 46, the relationship between past, present, and future selves does need to be addressed in rehabilitation practice and will be discussed in more depth in Chapter 5.

4.2.5 Achieving a good outcome

If the Samaritan had rubbed gravel instead of oil and wine into the wounds of the injured man he encountered he would not have been doing good, no matter how much compassion he felt. In fact he used a recognized method of caring for wounds that was well established in his culture. Not only that, after delegating further care to the innkeeper, he stated that when he returned he would check on the patient's progress and meet any associated costs.

Doing the good arises from right thinking and feeling, but is essentially about actions that have real as well as intended consequences. Moral behaviour is goal directed. After due consideration, we may make a good decision, but if that decision is not enacted, or if it is enacted but has unanticipated negative consequences we are not doing good. In order to do good we need to specify a desired outcome (itself not uncontroversial as we noted on p. 55), choose the course of action that is most likely to achieve it (other things being equal), check that the outcome has actually been achieved, and if necessary modify our actions. We also need to check that the desired outcome really is congruent with our moral values.

Practice principle 16. Use evidence-based interventions

Practice principle 17. Systematically monitor the degree to which your therapeutic objectives have been achieved

A simple example of this moral action system is given in Carver and Scheier's (1990) account of behavioural self-regulation (see also Carver and Scheier 1998; Baumeister and Exline 1999), and I develop it here. Suppose I hold to a basic principle arising from the moral value of beneficence—'be kind'. This may be expressed as a goal of keeping the pavement outside my home free of snow. This goal could be achieved by shovelling or sweeping the snow off the pavement. I give some thought to choosing the method that is most likely to be effective in removing the snow. I reflect on my own experience and I phone my father who is an expert on such things. On the basis of this evidence I decide that sweeping is the better method. I sweep the snow until it has been cleared to my satisfaction. I achieve my goal. But then I find, to my horror, that in removing the snow successfully I have exposed ice on the surface of the pavement. An elderly passer-by falls and is injured. This evidently violates the 'be kind' principle and forces me to rethink the whole enterprise.

This example makes the point that the behavioural goals I choose reflect the person I am trying to be (see Chapter 3). It is also likely that the method I choose to help me decide how to go about my goal will reflect something of who I am. In this example I place strong weight on someone I trust and whom I perceive as wise. Another person might have carried out an internet search or done a small experiment. In the next chapter we will discuss different approaches to the gathering and evaluation of evidence. For now it is important to note that there is less consensus in this area than one might expect.

4.2.6 Being good to myself

The example also illustrates the fact that a mismatch between the effect of our actions and our intentions can produce strong emotion. This is because our sense of who we are is not only *expressed by* our decisions, plans, and actions but *emerges from* them (Frankfurt 1971; Varela 1999). It is upsetting to find that I am carrying out harmful actions if I aspire to be a kind person, because through these actions I emerge as a careless and hurtful person. The close link between ethical behaviour and the sense of who I am is often expressed in the language of personal qualities or 'virtues' and 'vices', a way of approaching ethics that can be traced back to the ancient Greek philosopher, Aristotle. Personal ethics may be worked out around questions of the sort 'what would a prudent/kind/wise/compassionate person do in this situation?'

This sort of analysis locates morality in the person rather than in her action, and imparts a sense of personal responsibility for ethical decisions. It acknowledges that both ethical skills and technical skills are *personal* qualities, not merely cognitive behavioural patterns. Human beings learn many of our skills not through instruction, but through watching and copying others. We are particularly likely to copy those whom we admire. When people think through complex ethical dilemmas they may carry out a formal analysis of all the issues that is informed by rules and principles, but they are just as likely to ask 'What would X do?', particularly if X is a respected and more experienced friend or colleague. We think of someone we see as wise or compassionate and we try and act as if we too had those qualities. There is some evidence not only that working in teams facilitates this activity, but that wise decision making can be enhanced by it (Wertsch 1991; Staudinger and Baltes 1996).

Finally, this acknowledgement of the moral person as well as the moral action is important because it reminds us that we have a duty to look after ourselves—not just so that we are better able to contribute to the general good—'You'll be no use to anybody if you break down'—but because we see ourselves as worthwhile *for our own sakes*. This is something that is strongly emphasized by Kant, as we have seen (see p. 59), and implicit in the idea of loving your neighbour *as yourself*. Our own autonomy, agency, and well-being are important, and part of ethical practice is to care for ourselves.

We generally feel fulfilled and at ease in a situation where our behaviour, goals, and aspirations fit well with our sense of who we are or who we aspire to be (Higgins 2000). When there is a mismatch between what we are doing and striving towards and the way we see ourselves, we are likely to be anxious, unhappy, or dissatisfied (Sheldon and Kasser 1998). This holds true in the area of moral values (Camacho *et al.* 2003). If we work for an organization whose values are very different from our own we will find it hard to survive psychologically. Even where there is generally a good fit between our sense of who we are and our professional clinical practice, the nature of team decision making in ABI rehabilitation means that we will occasionally encounter a situation that requires us to go 'against the grain'. (In Chapter 1 the nurse who refused to help a patient to smoke was assertively expressing her values and feelings in this respect.) When this happens we will need to find a systematic way to manage the feelings that arise.

Practice principle 18. Aim for coherence between your professional practice and your sense of who you are

Practice principle 19. Be explicit about your personal values if relevant to the situation

Practice principle 20. Make clinical supervision that includes discussion of ethical aspects of practice an absolute priority

Clinical supervision is not an optional extra even for the most experienced of staff. Peer supervision, group supervision, or supervision from another professional can be particularly helpful when the question under discussion is ethical precisely because the wisdom required may be too great for any one person or any one perspective. The strong feelings that I have touched on in this chapter—empathy for our patients, guilt at having fallen short of our personal standards, indignation at injustice, anxiety because we don't know what to do for the best—mean that there is also a need for strong personal support, often more effective when it comes from peers than from superiors.

In this chapter I have presented 20 broad principles of ethical practice—doing the right thing—in ABI rehabilitation based on some approaches to living the good life. In the next chapter I will unpack some specific guidelines from each of them and begin to explore what doing good ABI rehabilitation might look like in more detail.

Suggestions for further reading

This is a range of texts that are either basic introductions to ethical theory and practice, more challenging but engaging essays on aspects of moral theory, or works on the psychology of virtue.

Bauman Z (1993). *Postmodern ethics*. Oxford, Blackwell.

Beauchamp T and Childress J (2002). *Principles of biomedical ethics*.
    Oxford, Oxford University Press.

Gilbert P (2005). *Compassion: conceptualisations, research and use in psychotherapy*.
    Hove, Routledge

Greene J, Sommerville B, Nystrom L, Darley J and Cohen J (2001). An fMRI investigation
    of emotional engagement in moral judgment. *Science* 293, 2105—2108.

Lévinas E (1981). *Otherwise than being*. London, Nijhoff.

May W (1994). The virtues in a professional setting. In K Fulford, H Gille and JM Soskice,
    eds. *Medical and moral reasoning*, pp. 75–90. Cambridge, Cambridge University Press.

Nussbaum M (1986). *The fragility of goodness*. Cambridge University Press, New York.

Nussbaum M (1990). *Love's knowledge*. Oxford University Press, New York.

Peterson C and Seligman M (2004). *Character strengths and virtues*.
    Oxford University Press, New York.

Ryan A (1993). *Justice*. Oxford University Press, Oxford.

Scruton R (2001). *Kant: a very short introduction*. Oxford University Press, Oxford.

Varela F (1999). *Ethical know-how: action, wisdom, and cognition*.
    Stanford University Press, Stanford CA.

References

Addington-Hall J and Kara L (2001). Measuring quality of life—who should measure
    quality of life? *British Medical Journal* **332**, 1417–1420.

Albrecht G and Devilieger P (1999). The disability paradox: high quality of life against all the odds. *Social Science and Medicine* **48**, 977–988.

Baddeley A (1998). The central executive: a concept and some misconceptions. *Journal of the International Neuropsychological Society* **4**, 523–526.

Bandura A (1999). Moral disengagement in the perpetration of inhumanities. *Social and Psychological Review* **3**, 193–209.

Bandura A, Barbaranelli C, Caprara G, Pastorelli C (1996). Mechanisms of moral disengagement in the exercise of moral agency. *Journal of Personality and Social Psychology* **71**, 364–374.

Banja J and Johnston M (1994). Outcomes evaluation in TBI rehabilitation: Part III: Ethical perspectives in social policy. *Archives of Physical Medicine and Rehabilitation* **75**, 19–25.

Barnard P and Teasdale J (1993). *Affect, cognition, and change.* Lawrence Erlbaum, Hove, East Sussex.

Bauman Z (1993). *Postmodern ethics.* Blackwell, Oxford.

Baumeister R (1987). How the self became a problem: A psychological review of historical research. *Journal of Personality and Social Psychology* **52**, 163–176.

Baumeister R and Exline J (1999). Virtue, personality and social relations: self-control as moral muscle. *Journal of Personality* **67**, 1165–1194.

Beauchamp T and Childress J (2001). *Principles of biomedical ethics.* Oxford University Press, Oxford.

Bernard J, Murphy M and Little M (1987). The failure of clinical psychologists to apply understood ethical principles. *Professional Psychology: Research and Practice* **18**, 489–491.

Brock D (1998). Ethical issues in the development of summary measures of health status. In *Summarising the population health: directions for the development and application of population metrics*, pp. 73–86. National Academy Press, Washington DC.

Burgess P, Alderman N, Evans J, Emslie H and Wislon B (1998). The ecological validity of tests of executive function. *Journal of the International Neuropsychological Society* **4**, 547–558.

Butler J (1999). *The ethics of health care rationing: principles and practices.* Cassell, London.

Camacho C, Higgins E and Luger L (2003). Moral value transfer from regulatory fit: what feels right is right and what feels wrong is wrong. *Journal of Personality and Social Psychology* **84**, 498–510.

Carr A, Gibson B and Robinson P (2002). Measuring quality of life. Is quality of life determined by expectation or experience? *British Medical Journal* **332**, 1240–1243.

Carver C and Scheier M (1990). Origins and function of positive and negative affect: a control process view. *Psychological Review* **97**, 19–36.

Carver C and Scheier M (1998). *On the self-regulation of behavior.* Cambridge University Press, New York.

Chan R (2001). Dysexecutive symptoms among a non-clinical sample. *British Journal of Psychology* **92**, 551–565.

Cookson R and Dolan P (2000). Principles of justice in health care rationing. *Journal of Medical Ethics* **26**, 323–329.

Confucius (2004). *Analects.* Translated by D Lau, Penguin, London.

Daniels N and Sabin J (2002). *Setting limits fairly: Can we learn to share medical resources?* Oxford University Press, Oxford.

Doyal L (1995). Needs, rights and equity: moral quality in healthcare rationing. *Quality in Health Care* **4**, 273–283.

Duncan J, Johnson R, Swales M and Freer C (1997). Frontal lobe deficits after head injury: unity and diversity of function. *Cognitive Neuropsychology* **14**, 713–741.

Farside B and Dunlop R (2001). Measuring quality of life: Is there such a thing as a life not worth living? *British Medical Journal* **322**, 1481–1483.

Finnis J (1993). Bland: Crossing the Rubicon? *Legal Quarterly Review* **109**, 329–337.

Fleming J, Tooth L, Hassell M and Chan W (1999). Prediction of community integration and vocational outcome 2–5 years after traumatic brain injury rehabilitation in Australia. *Brain Injury* **13**, 417–431.

Ford R and Richardson W (1994). Ethical decision making: a review of the empirical literature. *Journal of Business Ethics* **13**, 205–221.

Frankfurt H (1971). Freedom of the will and the concept of a person. *Journal of Philosophy* **68**, 5–20.

Guiton E (2002). How I learned to love life—even paralysed from the shoulders down. *The Guardian* 25 March, 1–2.

Harris J (1985). *The value of life*. Routledge, Abingdon.

Higgins E (2000). Making a good decision: value from fit. *American Psychologist* **55**, 1217–1230.

Janoff-Bulman R (1992). *Shattered assumptions: towards a new psychology of trauma*. Free Press, New York.

Jehn K (1994). Enhancing effectiveness: an investigation of advantages and disadvantages of value-based intragroup conflict. *International Journal of Conflict Management* **5**, 223–238.

Jehn K (1995). A multimethod examination of the benefits and detriments of intragroup conflict. *Administrative Science Quarterly* **40**, 256–282.

Kant I (1948/2005). *The moral law*. Translated by J Paton. Routledge, Abingdon.

Lepper M, Keavney M and Drake M (1996). Intrinsic motivation and extrinsic rewards: a commentary on Cameron and Pierce's meta-analysis. *Review of Educational Research* **66**, 5–32.

Macleod M and Smith J (2005). Gender and deprivation and rates of referral and thereby admission to a national neurorehabilitation service. *Clinical Rehabilitation* **19**, 1–7.

Malec J (1996). Ethical conflict resolution based on an ethic of relationship for brain injury rehabilitation. *Brain Injury* **10**, 781–795.

Matthews M (1987). Codes of ethics: organizational behaviour and misbehaviour. *Research in Corporate Social Performance* **9**, 107–130.

McGrath J and King N (2004). Acquired brain injury. In J Bennett-Levy, G Butler, M Fennell, A Hackmann, M Mueller and D Westbrook, eds. *The Oxford guide to behavioural experiments in cognitive therapy*, pp. 337–339. Oxford University Press, Oxford.

Murray C and Acharya A (1997). Understanding DALYs. *Journal of Health Economics* **16**, 703–730.

National Institute for Health and Clinical Excellence (2005). *Social value judgements: principles for the development of NICE guidance*. http://www.nice.org.uk/page.aspx?o=svjguidance [accessed 1.8.06].

Nord E (1999). *Cost-value analysis in health care: making sense out of QALYs.* Cambridge University Press, Cambridge.

Padesky C and Greenberger D (1995). *Clinician's guide to mind over mood.* Guilford, New York.

Parkin A (1998). The central executive does not exist. *Journal of the International Neuropsychological Society* **4**, 518–522.

Rosenthal M and Lourie I (1996). Ethical issues in the evaluation of competence in persons with acquired brain injuries. *Neurorehabilitation* **6**, 113–121.

Scott R (1998). *Professional ethics: a guide for rehabilitation professionals.* Mosby, St Louis, MO.

Sheldon K and Kasser (1998). Pursuing personal goals: skills enable progress but not all progress is beneficial. *Personality and Social Psychology Bulletin* **24**, 1319–1331.

Staudinger U and Baltes P (1996). Interactive minds: a facilitative setting for wisdom-related performance. *Journal of Personality and Social Psychology* **71**, 746–762.

Swiercinsky D (2002). Ethical issues in neuropsychological rehabilitation. In S Bush and M Drexler, eds. *Ethical issues in clinical neuropsychology*, pp. 135–163. Swets and Zeitlinger, Lisse.

Varela F (1999). *Ethical know-how: action, wisdom, and cognition.* Stanford University Press, Stanford CA.

Vetlessen AJ (1993). Why does proximity make a moral difference? *Praxis International* **12**, 371–386.

Wade D (1999). Goal planning in stroke rehabilitation: How? *Topics in Stroke Rehabilitation* **6**, 16–36.

Watts F (2004). Christian theology. In F Watts and E Gulliford, eds. *Forgiveness in context: theology and psychology in creative dialogue*, pp. 50–68. Continuum, London.

Wertsch J (1991). *Voices of the mind: a sociocultural approach to mediated action.* Harvard University Press, Cambridge MA.

Wilson T and Dunn E (2003). Self-knowledge: its limits, value, and potential for improvement. *Annual Review of Psychology* **55**, 493–518.

Chapter 5

Ethical rehabilitation practice

On p. 47 I stated that the aim of rehabilitation is to support the person with acquired brain injury (ABI) in establishing a new sense of identity continuous with, but not stuck in, the past, while managing the medical complications, pain, and emotional distress that arise during the process. Background or setting conditions can sustain and nurture the sort of good, and thus ethical, practice that is necessary for this process. This chapter begins with a brief consideration of these conditions before moving on to specify detailed guidelines under each of the ethical practice principles generated in Chapter 4.

5.1 Setting conditions: compassion, wisdom, and hope

Virtues and vices are usually thought of as attributes of individual persons and, as discussed on p. 73, this has clear benefits. However, it is also possible and useful to consider virtues and vices as characteristics of systems or groups of persons ('institutional racism' and 'national pride' are obvious examples), and the following discussion refers to both individual practitioners and the organizations within which they work.

The three cardinal virtues in healthcare practice are compassion, wisdom, and hope. I have already explored compassion at length in Chapter 4. It is the foundation for the whole healthcare enterprise. But good practice also requires wisdom, and should be carried out in a culture that inspires hope.

5.1.1 Wisdom

Wisdom is essentially practical knowledge (Baltes and Staudinger 2000)— knowing how to approach the situations characterized by novelty, complexity, or partial knowledge that are so familiar to ABI practitioners. Wisdom is traditionally associated with experience. A good amount of previous relevant experience decreases the novelty factor in challenging clinical situations. However, this is about more than the 'I've seen it all before' boast of the old hand. The sort of experience that may be most important in the development of clinical wisdom is the wrestling with hard questions that are thrown up by difficult situations. This active participation is conducive to the development of both the cognitive skills and emotional resilience necessary to deal with them effectively. The presence of experienced practitioners in rehabilitation teams (or at least access to the insights of experienced practitioners) is likely to improve the rate of good decisions that are made.

One recent analysis of wisdom (Linley 2004) identifies three essential features:

1. Integration of cognition and affect.

2. Recognition and acceptance of limitation.

3. Tolerating uncertainty and ambiguity.

These are easily applied to the clinical situation. First, the integration of cognition and affect (or in the terms of the discussion on p. 69 'heart' and 'head') relates closely to the argument in Chapter 4 that rational ethical systems need to be held together with emotional moral impulses in directing what is right. Secondly, the recognition of and acceptance of limitation is a key component of the process of balancing high ideals and aspirations for clinical services with the realities of limited resources, knowledge, and available options, also identified in Chapter 4. Thirdly, the ability to tolerate uncertainty and ambiguity is necessary in an enterprise where the prognosis for each patient is uncertain at multiple levels, and where therapeutic goals may therefore be equally uncertain. Therapeutic goals are themselves central to the establishment and maintenance of hope (Snyder 1994; Snyder *et al* 1996), the final setting condition for good rehabilitation practice.

5.1.2 Hope

Hope is at the heart of all healthcare, and is clearly especially important in situations that appear hopeless (Snyder 1995). As discussed in Chapter 3, because the situation in ABI can often appear hopeless a positive therapeutic approach that encourages hope is extremely important (Adams 1996; Elliott and Kurylo 2000; McGrath 2004; Siegert *et al* 2004; Collicutt McGrath and Linley 2006). The person with ABI is hoping to resume some sort of normal life, to re-establish, maintain, and develop a sense of identity and worth. In Chapter 3 we saw that goals are important in contributing to this sense of identity and worth, punctuating personal narratives, organizing habitual behaviours, and springing from personal values. Actively taking the patient's goals into account is therefore a key part of the enterprise of rehabilitation.

Focusing rehabilitation on goals to be achieved rather than problems to be overcome keeps the process positive and constructive, rather than negative and corrective (Seligman 2002; Ward and Brown 2004). But it is also crucial to understand that, as with us all, the person with ABI does not need so much to have achieved the goal—to be there, as to be making good progress towards the goal—to be securely on the way there. This is another way of stating the cliché that to journey is as important as to arrive at the destination. But there is more. The destination itself may not be entirely clear for much of the journey.

Rehabilitation professionals are well used to tolerating fuzzy rehabilitation aims, especially where these involve 'horizon goals.'[1] For example, a rehabilitation team may tell a patient with perfect literal honesty that he is participating in a programme designed to 'support him in return to work at an appropriate level'. Everything hangs of course on how one understands 'support', 'work', 'appropriate', and 'level'. The team has left the wording vague in order to hold together the potential discrepancy between the professionals' and the patient's vision for the future, so that the rehabilitation process may proceed smoothly. This sort of practice can feel dishonest, and hence unethical. It can also feel insufficiently focused and specific, and hence unprofessional.

But that instinct of setting fuzzy horizon goals is a good instinct. This is for three reasons. First, as already discussed, the outcome is often uncertain in ABI rehabilitation. In very many cases professionals genuinely cannot be certain what they are aiming at, especially in the longer term.

Secondly, horizon goals are by their nature fuzzy for all of us. They only come into focus as we get close to them. We know what we want to do today in very specific terms, what we want to do next month in more general terms, what we want to do next year in more vague terms yet, and what we want out of life as a whole in fuzzy terms. While our immediate goals are focused and *urgent*, our horizon goals are fuzzy but *important*[2] because they provide the directional compass for all that we do.

Thirdly, some philosophers (for example Dewey 1922/2002) and proponents of chaos theory (for example Gleick 1988) argue that, as we approach the horizon, our horizon goals come into focus not because they have been there waiting all the time for us to get close enough to see them, but instead *emerge from the act of moving towards them*. There is a sense in which we create these sorts of goals *from* our actions. We grope in a certain broad direction, and the groping becomes progressively more refined until its goal is realized. Yet the goal has in some rudimentary sense been present within the action all the time. So, our patient participating in a work rehabilitation programme and the professionals working with him are both groping in the same broad direction, and the final outcome will emerge *from* their joint activity, it does not exist in advance of it. They are therefore correct, not dishonest, to state the horizon goal at the outset in broad and fuzzy terms, but with the hope and intention of eventual refinement.

This understanding of horizon goals as important, but emergent from dynamic action as opposed to preformed and fixed before any action is undertaken, helps

---

[1] I am grateful to Dr Duncan Babbage for this term, which he uses to describe ultimate life aspirations as opposed to discharge goals.

[2] See Hope and Butler (1995, pp. 37–38) for a discussion of the difference between the urgent and important.

us to understand how the present can be invested with hope as opposed to worry or despair. If the horizon goal is inherent in the action then the present moment is important and full of meaning (rehabilitation activities are experienced as creative and personally owned). If the horizon goal lies somewhere outside the action at some distant point, then the present can either become enslaved to the future, (rehabilitation activities are experienced as 'doing time' until real life is resumed) or disconnected from the future altogether, losing all direction and meaning (rehabilitation activities are experienced as pointless and dehumanizing).

The commitment to future-as-project is one of the conditions for the emergence or re-emergence of a sense of self (Alexander 1987, p. 135; Hooker 1999). So, recovering ABI patients, perhaps more than any other group, need to feel that they are on the way somewhere. Rehabilitation professionals should provide clear local markers of progress along the way (for instance 'SMART' objectives—see Practice principle 17), clearly connect these with an ultimate destination, but tolerate a broad and fuzzy description of this ultimate destination. In this they will be doing something quite profound: treating their patients like human beings (rather than objects on a production line), the first practice principle to which we now turn.

5.2 **Putting guidelines into practice**

5.2.1 **Practice principle 1. Despite some appearances to the contrary, people with ABI are human persons and should be treated as such**

On p. 38 I outlined four ways of treating a patient like a human being. The first involves behaving towards the patient as if he is sentient and has some coherent mental life:

- ◆ do not talk to others about him in his presence without also addressing him
- ◆ use eye contact and appropriately
- ◆ observe the usual social courtesies of greeting
- ◆ assume that the patient is able to feel pain and discomfort and manage this appropriately.

The second involves treating the patient's body parts as essential aspects of a whole human being:

- ◆ observe the usual requirements of physical and personal privacy and boundaries appropriate to the patient's culture
- ◆ ask permission throughout acts of physical care giving, or if the patient is unable to respond inform her of what you are doing throughout the procedure.

The third involves supporting the patient's agency. This will be discussed in detail later in this chapter under Practice Principle 3. The final way involves treating the patient as a social being by making a relationship with him. This in its turn depends on empathy, seeing the patient as a human person *like me but at the same time distinct from me*. This can be divided into seeing the *previous person*, seeing the *real person*, seeing the *aspirational person*, and seeing the *whole person*.

Ways that can help us to see the *previous person* include:

- looking at photographs of the patient taken before her injury
- carrying out a systematic exploration of the patient's previous roles and relationships, always remembering that these are very often perceived by the patient as continuing roles and relationships (take care to ask, 'What *is* your job', not 'What *was* your job?')
- identifying, locating, and reading any advance directives

Seeing the *real person* can be difficult. Often our patients seem like blank canvases for us to paint as we see fit, especially if they are not easily able to communicate with us, thereby disconfirming our projections. Cultural and ethnic differences can lead us to project stereotypical qualities on to our patients. For instance: a 'posh' English accent may call up the judgement 'snob'; an adolescent grunt may call up the judgement 'yob'; an unfamiliar ethnic accent or language may call up the judgement 'strange' or 'uncivilized'; a body covered in tattoos may call up the judgement 'violent.' We are also apt to project idealized qualities such as bravery, patience, and wisdom on to people whom we perceive as suffering, weak, and vulnerable. (I discovered this tendency in myself when I ran a news discussion group for patients I thought I knew well and whom I thought I liked, only to find that many of them expressed sexist, racist, and reactionary political views. I had seen 'sick person' and conflated this with 'saint' (Sargent *et al.* 2000).)

Ways that can help us to see the *real person* include:

- Carrying out a systematic exploration of the patient's current tastes, preferences, beliefs, and values, and the wider culture from which they have emerged
- Respecting her right to hold her values and beliefs even where these are different from or offensive to our own (instead of trying to like the patient by projecting our own views on to her)
- Going beyond personality descriptions or diagnostic labels to explain behaviour ('She lies in bed because she is lazy', 'He asks for China tea because he is a snob', 'He won't participate in therapy because he is passive', 'He shouts at visitors on the ward because he is aggressive', 'She never complains because she is brave', 'He won't leave his room because he is

psychotic', 'He keeps phoning prostitutes because he is disinhibited') and instead asking how the behaviour relates to the patient's values and previous and current life aspirations

The *aspirational person* is a person with hopes for the future. These hopes may or may not have been modified by the experience of ABI. It is likely that horizon goals will remain largely unchanged. Unless the patient is in total denial, more proximal goals, or at least the time-scales within which these operate, will have been reappraised. For instance, a law student may still hope to become a solicitor but may defer active pursuit of this goal until she has learnt to walk again. Ways that can help us see the aspirational person include:

- carrying out a systematic exploration of both his proximal and his horizon goals. Understanding each goal in itself and also the way proximal goals are linked to horizon goals can go a long way towards explaining behaviour. ('She lies in bed because she is afraid of falling and impeding her recovery', 'He asks for China tea because it is a way of reminding himself who he is', 'He won't participate in therapy because it doesn't connect with his planned lifestyle after discharge', 'He shouts at visitors on the ward because he is overstimulated and can't remove himself to a quiet place', 'She never complains because thinks she will get out more quickly if she is compliant', 'He won't leave his room because he wants to avoid other patients he thinks are out to get him', 'He keeps phoning prostitutes because he is worried about his identity and worth as a man, and sexual relations with women are his way of defining this')

Finally, ways that help us see the *whole person* include:

- seeing the patient in his own environment (visiting his home or place of work)
- seeing the patient in her own clothes, not exclusively in the tracksuit and trainer uniform of many rehabilitation units
- meeting the patient's friends and family
- seeing the patient in a setting where the dominant agenda is not the tasks of rehabilitation—sharing leisure or 'play' with the patient

The way in which the guidelines presented in this section are actually implemented will vary with the particular rehabilitation service and the characteristics of the service users. The first six are non-negotiable. Not all of the others will be achievable by every service. Some of them will be easier to implement in long-stay residential units, others in community-based out-patient services. Some can be implemented by single practitioners, but they more naturally fit a team approach. The system developed at Rivermead Rehabilitation Centre in the 1990s contains many of these components, including a questionnaire and structured interview that explores previous roles, current values, proximal goals, and horizon goals, together with an occupational therapy led service targeting leisure for its own sake (Wade 1999). Practitioners have found that the use of the Rivermead Life Goals Questionnaire, if nothing else, helps them to 'see' in greater depth the patients they thought they knew—to enter into the patient's perspective, and thus to empathize.

5.2.2 Practice principle 2. Don't make things worse

People with ABI are in a situation full of losses and potential losses. But it is possible for practitioners to make things even worse, either inadvertently or in pursuit of some higher goal that may be invoked to justify their actions. Operating outside the limits of one's competence risks making things worse. Operating at the edge of one's competence without supervision risks making things worse:

- If you have not had training or achieved an acceptable degree of competence in a procedure do not carry it out, even if the procedure might help the patient's situation.

- If you have had training but are at the limit of your competence in a procedure only carry it out under supervision, even if the procedure might help the patient's situation.

Encountering a bad situation can put professionals into a 'something must be done' frame of mind. This is not always a good idea, and is an example of where strong emotion can lead to bad decisions. Doing something could make a bad situation worse (for instance taking action that could alert the perpetrator where a vulnerable adult is being abused before arrangements can be made to remove her to a safe place):

- Carry out a risk assessment so that unwanted effects of a proposed course of action can be anticipated and contingency action plans formulated. If the risks look too great consider the 'do nothing' option.

Sometimes nothing can be done. It is in situations like these that experienced practitioners may need to give others permission to do nothing, and help deal with the feelings of unprofessionalism, frustration, and regret that may go along with such decisions.

- But do not use the 'do nothing' option as an excuse to evade difficult decisions. This sort of judgement is something to be discussed in supervision sessions.

The practice of making things worse on purpose so that they can eventually get better is quite common in healthcare. An example in the rehabilitation setting is the serial plastering of contracted limbs (which causes discomfort and often pain) in order to increase range of movement with a view to achieving standing and walking. Another example is inflicting pain or removing privileges as part of a programme aimed at improving social behaviour and re-integrating the patient into the community. These sorts of procedures should always be viewed critically and the following questions asked:

- How likely is the procedure to be successful in achieving the desired goal?
- Is there an alternative less aversive means of achieving the same or similar goal?
- Is the goal something that the patient wants?
- Does the patient understand and has she consented to the procedure?

Only if the goal is desired by the patient, the procedure is understood and consented to[3] by the patient, and there is no effective alternative, should procedures that make things worse in order to make them better be considered. This means that more often than not there will be a decision not to implement such procedures. (Certainly there have been great advances in behavioural methodology that have rendered aversive and punitive approaches to behavioural control obsolete on practical grounds alone (Rothwell *et al.* 1999). The situation with physical treatments remains more complex.)

The situation is complicated when the patient agrees to the goal but not to the aversive means necessary to achieve it. In some ways this is not very different from the general human phenomenon expressed, for example, in a longing to be slim alongside the tendency to put off dieting and exercise indefinitely. If the team suspects that the problem here is related to cognitive impairment—perhaps an acquired difficulty with linking means to ends—then psychological approaches to improving cognitive self-regulation (Hart and Evans 2006) should certainly be attempted. But if these do not produce a change of heart the choice of the individual needs to be respected.

5.2.3 Practice principle 3. Promote the agency, distinctive identity, and freedom of the patient

In Chapter 3 human agency, distinctive identity and freedom of were discussed at length. The guidelines in this section follow from that discussion.

- Find out what name the person likes to be called (this may bear no obvious relation to the name on her medical notes) and use it—try and spell it correctly.
- Ensure the maintenance of psychological boundaries by treating personal information about the patient with discretion, and as confidential within

---

[3] The issue of informed consent will be discussed in detail under Practice principle 11.

the immediate clinical team. (This point is discussed in more detail under Practice principle 7.)

♦ Promote free and independent movement and action, giving physical and psychological support to the patient in accord with her physical and psychological abilities.

♦ Do not use physical restraint and restriction (for instance applying wheel-chair brakes, locking doors) as means to manage problem behaviour.

♦ Ensure that the immediate physical and psychosocial environment does not restrict his liberty through poor signposting, orientating features, or physical obstacles.

♦ Support attempts to minimize constraints in the wider environment by modification to home and work environment, provision of physical and psychological aids, etc.

♦ Support the patient in constructing a personal narrative of her life and fitting recent events into this narrative. This narrative will need to be documented in writing or on audiotape, particularly if the patient has memory problems, so that she can return to it repeatedly. If the patient has communication problems use pictures and drawings to supplement or replace words. The narrative will include the language of events, personality traits, motives, emotions, and goals.

♦ Where possible give the patient a sense of being in control of his mental life. Acknowledge your own mistakes when you make them. If the patient's account of reality is very distorted find ways of acknowledging the patient's *feelings* and sidestep active collusion with his thinking. Do not constantly draw attention to the mistakes the patient makes in order to instil 'insight'. You are more likely to instil a sense of failure and discouragement. Treat rehabilitation as a process of building skills rather than removing faults.

♦ Find out what the patient's proximal goals and wishes are. (In other words what he wants in the immediate future and what he hopes to get out of rehabilitation.) *Remember the patient is the expert on how he feels and what he wants.* Formally acknowledge the patient's wishes even if they are unrealistic or it is not possible to deliver them. This gives the patient a voice.

♦ Where possible build at least something of what the patient wants into her treatment plan. (This is unfortunately still not standard practice in Britain at least (Holliday *et al.* 2005).) Share the plan with the patient. Give her a permanent record, in writing in her own language or in pictorial or symbolic form as appropriate. The plan should not just refer to task performance but also to things that give the patient pleasure or cultural affirmation such as access to preferred food, clothing, or religious space.

+ Use the knowledge you have obtained from your systematic exploration of the patient's previous roles and relationships, current tastes, preferences, beliefs, values, and culture (p. 83) to formulate horizon goals collaboratively.

Often a patient's proximal goals are unrealistic (for instance 'being able to walk independently') but his horizon goal is reasonable ('to continue to be a good father to my son'). These goals may be linked by cultural and personal beliefs ('good dads play football with their sons'). Much work then needs to be carried out in disconnecting the unrealistic proximal goal from the horizon goal and substituting an alternative ('being able to play computer games or table football'). For a more extensive discussion of this process see McGrath and Adams (1999).

5.2.4 Practice principle 4. Think outside the box: your moral responsibility may extend further than you thought

There are many advantages to team working. They include peer support, the opportunity to share wisdom and apply multiple perspectives, and the capacity for the whole to be more than the sum of its parts. But there are also disadvantages. It is possible to be a passenger, to sit back and let others do the bulk of the work. It also means that clinical and moral responsibility is hard to pin down. It is easy to make excuses such as 'it's not my role', 'it was a team decision— don't blame me', and so on.

+ If you are involved in an interdisciplinary team contribute actively to the *team process* not just your own professional area.

+ Where decisions and actions fall outside the clear remit of any one profession consider taking responsibility for them. If you lack confidence or competence collaborate with another team member.

+ Take some responsibility for the whole process and system of rehabilitation in your service. Use existing means or establish new means to comment and propose change or consolidation (for instance a service 'away day').

Sometimes service innovations can result from a broadening of perspective and a seizing of moral responsibility. In the early 1990s I found myself becoming increasingly aware of the children of patients in my unit. I was particularly struck by two children of a young woman who had sustained a severe traumatic brain injury and who was behaviourally unpredictable, dysphasic, and confused. I often noticed them running about on the unit having been brought along by grandparents to visit. They appeared perplexed and frightened by the things they saw. I found myself wondering what sense they made of their mother's situation. I felt bad that there was nothing for them to do and no safe or familiar place for them to go. I wondered if it would be better for them not to visit at all. I wondered how one might explain their mother's problems to them. I wondered how they were feeling. I thought my nursing or social work colleagues should do something about it. I approached them, and while they were very sympathetic, were not in a position to take any action. Eventually I decided that *I* should do something. I managed to obtain agreement for the development of a clinical psychology service to the children of our patients, initially only one session a week. In 1995 a clinical psychologist was appointed. Since then she has built up not only an excellent small service, but just as importantly a body of knowledge and resources for the children of parents with brain injury (Daisley 2002; Webster and Daisley 2005). The impetus for this seizing of the moral initiative and taking of clinical responsibility was my *emotional* reaction to the expressions on the faces of two children (see next section).

Moral responsibility may also extend to campaigning for the provision and safeguarding of services for a particular client group. An example is the case of Mrs Pat Morris, a nurse who left her job to seek a judicial review in relation to Trafford Healthcare NHS Trust. The Trust had closed two rehabilitation wards without going through a process of public consultation. In September 2006 the High Court ruled that the closure was illegal, and in response the NHS Trust initiated a *post hoc* public consultation process. Mrs Morris was awarded costs. She clearly felt that, despite the financial risk, it was her moral duty to take action in this way.

5.2.5 Practice principle 5. Welcome and make proper use of empathic and other emotion as a basis for moral action

Empathic emotion is called up when we have come close enough to another person to feel what happens to him in some way as happening to us.

- Reflect on your feelings of empathy. Do they arise from an accurate understanding or are you just projecting your own issues on to the patient? It is more likely that the empathy is genuine if the patient is generally unlike you. You are in more danger of projecting your issues if the patient is close to you in age and gender or if something in the patient's situation resonates with an issue in your own life.

- Where you find it hard to empathize is it because the patient is just too different from you for you to be able to make a genuine connection? Or is it that the patient's situation touches on painful issues in your own life that you would rather avoid?

- Use your feelings of empathy as a way to alert yourself and others to issues that you might have overlooked.

Feelings of unease can alert us to ethical conflicts.

- Tune into your feelings of unease or disquiet. Try and make clear to yourself what it is that is making you uneasy. It is likely to be a conflict between a proposed course of action, or something you have done, and a moral principle or value. Get used to saying 'I am not comfortable with …' as a means of opening up a conversation about the issues with yourself or others.

- Reflecting on feelings takes time and effort. It often happens after a critical event. Be realistic and make time to do this. Consider keeping a feelings journal alongside clinical note keeping.

5.2.6 Practice principle 6. Acknowledge the emotional experience of the patient and address any emotional distress

Rehabilitation has traditionally been about task performance. Where the emotions of patients are considered this is often because they are seen as getting in the way of the main agenda—improved behavioural function. However, the subjective emotional feelings of patients are important in their own right. As we establish empathy with a patient this becomes obvious. The narrative and goal focused approaches described in previous sections include within them an explicit acknowledgement and recording of the patient's feelings, and may be sufficient to address emotional needs. But there are other things that can be done:

- Much emotion expressed by patients is normal given their situation. Reassurance of this normality can be very helpful.

- Much emotion expressed by patients is positive. Encourage its expression and enjoy sharing it with them.

- Much distress is caused by poor communication, especially regarding progress. Providing appropriate written or pictorial information can be very helpful.

- Some distress is inevitable because some situations cannot be changed. Provide a private and safe place for the expression of emotion.

- The patient's usual means of coping with distress may no longer be available. Help her think through alternative strategies (for instance, playing a relaxation tape instead of going for a jog, painting a picture instead of talking to friends).

- Identify local or regional sources of specialist help or advice if distress is severe and persistent or stops the person from functioning.

5.2.7 Practice principle 7. Take all interested parties into account

In addition to the patient, interested parties may include:

- family (including children)
- friends
- neighbours
- employers
- other service users
- members of the clinical team
- other staff members (including administrative and domestic staff)
- staff from statutory and voluntary community services who are likely to come in contact with the patient
- members of the general public who are likely to come in contact with the patient
- funding bodies and insurers
- officers of the law.

Thankfully, not all of these will be relevant in every case. Special care should be taken not to overlook the interests of 'invisible' people such as children, domestic staff, and staff who only work night shifts. It is also important to acknowledge that the members of the clinical team caring for the patient are interested parties in their own right. As part of the process of clinical decision making their cultural, professional, and moral values should be treated with respect, and their physical and psychological well-being safeguarded.

A systematic means of assessing and recording the expectations and needs of family members is an important part of the rehabilitation process (see for instance the Rivermead Relatives' Expectations and Wishes Questionnaire; Wade 1999). It is not only patients who may have unrealistic expectations. There may also be a mismatch between the patient's hopes and expectations and that of other family members (for instance concerning final place of residence), and it is important to identify such mismatches at the earliest possible point. Family members may be under emotional or financial stress, and sources of emotional support and practical advice should be identified for them. Local branches of voluntary agencies such as Headway,[4]

---

[4] Headway, 4 King Edward Court, King Edward Street, Nottingham NG1 1EW, UK. http://www.headway.org.uk

The Stroke Association,[5] Different Strokes,[6] and carer support groups can be invaluable.

Making sure that all interested parties are in the 'communication loop' while safeguarding the privacy of the patient is extremely challenging. Individual clinicians can wield enormous and inappropriate power by being the sole repositories of certain key facts about the patient under the guise of maintaining confidentiality. Equally, teams can enter into feeding frenzies of clinical gossip exchange about every sort of detail of the patient's life.

It is good practice for a small core team, whose composition will vary depending on the situation of the patient and the type of services involved, to hold all the clinical and psychosocial information, and to share this with others on a 'need to know' basis. This begs the question 'need to know for what purpose?' Information sharing protocols can be very helpful in this situation. These protocols should be informed by national guidelines (e.g. the NHS Code of Practice on Confidentiality 2003) and the law (e.g. the Data Protection Act 1998). They need to list all interested parties; to have some indication of what information each interested party needs to know and why; to document which individuals hold information; to include regularly updated evidence that the patient has agreed to the sharing of relevant information with family members, social care agencies, or employers. It is also important for the patient to know who holds information about her, and some procedure for keeping the patient informed should be included on this sort of protocol. Above all it should be short and user-friendly.

A single multidisciplinary report for distribution to health and social care agencies and other interested parties can greatly aid communication, especially at transition points such as discharge from in-patient care. It is, however, important that detailed sensitive personal information is not included in these sorts of reports. Rather, a source for more information in various areas (e.g. 'family situation', 'financial situation') should be specified.

There are some situations in which information should be shared with others against the wishes of the patient. These are where abuse or serious harm can be prevented by disclosing the information, or where the investigation of a crime would be advanced through the sharing of information. Here the interests of the general public or specific others are judged to outweigh the interests of the patient with regard to privacy.

---

5 Stroke Association, 240 City Road, London EC1V 2PR, UK. http://www.stroke.org.uk

6 Different Strokes, 9 Canon Harnett Court, Wolverton Mill, Milton Keynes MK12 5NF, UK. http://www.differentstrokes.co.uk

5.2.8 **Practice principle 8. Be realistic about available resources**

This principle follows on from, and blends into the previous one, because taking all interested parties into account has implications for the fair distribution of resources. While it is important always to bear in mind that resources are limited when delivering a rehabilitation service, thought should also be given to how resources may be increased and safeguarded (see Practice principle 4), and to how they can be managed through cost-effective practice. For this reason it is extremely important that the efficacy and efficiency of therapeutic interventions are critically evaluated. (see discussion under Practice principle 16).

Waiting lists for assessment, admission, and treatment should be run according to agreed principles that are set out in writing, and accessible to all interested parties. The principles for managing the waiting list may vary depending on the nature of the service. They are likely to combine an ethical utilitarian principle with practical considerations. For instance the principle may be 'Other things being equal, first come first served.' The 'Other things' to be taken into consideration could include the annual leave pattern of a staff member with specialist skills in the area needed by the patient or the availability of a necessary piece of specialist equipment at the time. Alternatively, one could devise two waiting lists operating according to principles of 'urgent' and 'important'—the 'urgent' list moving faster but the 'important' list being safeguarded in some way so that it did not grind to a halt. Patients could be triaged and assigned to either list. An example of an urgent situation would be a mother who had sustained a stroke during the process of childbirth. Rehabilitation aimed at helping her form a physical and emotional bond with her baby is much less likely to be successful if started late after a long period of mother–child separation. An example of an important situation is the neuropsychological reassessment of a man 5 years after he has sustained a head injury to help him with future career planning. It needs to be done, but it could probably wait a few months without undue detriment.

Time-limited interventions should also be considered. These are easier to deliver in the later stages of rehabilitation. In the earlier stages change is so rapid and outcome so uncertain that specifying the content and duration of treatment programmes in advance is not always appropriate. Nevertheless, while rehabilitation is a conceptually open-ended process, in practical terms specific courses of treatment come to an end. This culture needs to be made clear to patients and relatives from the start. Most ABI rehabilitation services in the USA and some in the UK offer only pre-specified time limited programmes. But many British services have more discretion, and ethical decisions concerning when to bring treatment to an end are devolved to individual practitioners.

Because it always seems as if more can be done it often feels difficult to bring individually tailored courses of treatment to an end. The end of therapy (which includes the end of a therapeutic relationship) emphasizes the fact that the patient has reached a point where significant improvement is no longer expected. Patients often complain at the use of the term 'plateau'—'There is no point having any more sessions because you have plateaued.' A plateau is a flat plain at the top of a mountain. The patient climbs the mountain of recovery, reaches a plateau and no more hope is left. This does not do justice to the process of recovery after brain injury, which is more like a series of ups and downs with a generally upward trend that becomes less steep, *but does not stop*, as time goes on.

The end of treatment should not be presented as an individual clinical decision, arrived at late in the day and based on a judgement about the patient's potential for change, because this can feel like a decision based on a kind of clinical 'deservingness'. 'It's not worth it' is often heard as 'You're not worth it.' Time-limited treatments should be presented at the outset on the basis of their cost-effective nature in managing limited resources in a service that aims to offer the maximum number of patients 'good enough' courses of treatment. The fact that resources are limited should be honestly presented as a fact of life. The fact that progress can be expected for many years should also be acknowledged. The time-limited treatment should be presented as the best that this service can offer you at this point in your recovery, no more or less than others are getting, perhaps less than ideal.

The process of setting rehabilitation goals should express this. First the horizon goals should be acknowledged and related to the present situation, but it must be made clear that horizon goals may not be attained within the present course of treatment; further work may need to be done by other services or by this service at a future point. (For instance it is right to acknowledge that a patient wants to resume her old employment. It is right to work on a programme aimed at independent walking as a prerequisite for this, ensuring that the walking skills learnt are appropriate to her work-related activities. But this does not mean that the programme can necessarily continue uninterrupted until she achieves a return to work.) Secondly, the wording of more immediate goals should include a time frame (see Practice principle 17). Treatment may end when either this time has passed or when the goals have been achieved, depending on the service.

Finally, a service may decide to specialize in only one type of patient, perhaps those with predominantly psychological problems, or those with predominantly physical problems. Or it may choose to carry out only those interventions that have easily measured outcomes. The composition of the clinical team would then reflect the skill mix appropriate to the interventions concerned.

This is one way of managing limited resources that may be appealing in the short term, but it is a significant move away from the patient-centred practice described in Chapter 3 because it offers a partitioned or fragmented service, rather than a holistic service (Banja 1994). People with ABI rarely have exclusively psychological or exclusively physical needs, especially in the early stages of recovery. Only acknowledging or responding to some of the patient's current needs is in conflict with Practice principle 1 and may also be less cost-effective in the long term. To quote a commentator on the situation in the USA, '... brain injury rehabilitation ... has been squelched for the sake of short-term economics.' (Swiercinsky 2002).

5.2.9 Practice principle 9. Use, and if necessary develop, practice standards and protocols to temper emotion

We have considered practice standards already under Practice principles 7 and 8.

In these contexts transparent protocols are used to make clear to all interested parties that practice in a complex situation involving conflicting interests has been uniform and fair.

Written practice standards and protocols are also useful to give clinicians an alternative more 'objective' perspective in situations where they have become personally involved. They can remind the team of agreed principles that they have forgotten because other things appear more compelling and salient. An example would be the right of a patient to make a 'bad' decision. This is a principle that may be accepted in theory, but which a team ignores when it sees a patient getting into an undesirable relationship. The emotional instinct to care can be overwhelming. An example from the Rivermead goal planning protocols is the principle to postpone a scheduled goal planning meeting if information about the patient's wishes and expectancies is not available. In this situation the temptation to proceed on the basis of guessing what the patient wants is almost overwhelming, given time pressures and the great inconvenience of rescheduling interdisciplinary meetings. But the rule was drawn up because it was found that decisions taken on the basis of guesses often had to be revoked later, and an additional meeting organized anyway.

In both these examples the protocols give teams permission to take a 'hands off' approach. They replace the lower level professional instinct to act responsibly, by taking protective action or not wasting time, with a higher authority that says 'Wait!' In this respect protocols can act rather like a cognitive 'central executive', inhibiting habitual or stimulus bound behaviour and taking wider consideration into account.

Conversely protocols can be vital energizers of behaviour in situations where teams may be uncertain what to do and therefore at risk of doing nothing, for instance when there is a vague suspicion of abuse of a vulnerable adult (see for instance Department of Health and Home Office Guidance 2000) or child (Department of Health Circular 2003). Locally drawn up child protection and vulnerable adult policies emphasize the need for appropriate action, specify a chain of responsibility (whom to contact), and explain where other considerations such as confidentiality can be overridden. The regular review and refinement of these sorts of protocols makes them repositories of accumulative wisdom.

5.2.10 **Practice principle 10. Do not be enslaved to practice standards and protocols**

The principles for drawing up practice standards and protocols are likely to have been formulated by national bodies. But local situations are likely to be highly variable. Therefore the drawing up of local guidelines will depend on good knowledge of the local situation and how this relates to more general principles of good practice. Local situations are likely to change fairly rapidly, especially with regard to staff who are in post. Therefore guidelines should be updated regularly. National guidelines cannot just be taken on board wholesale.

Often local guidelines specify the minimum that is required—what a service needs to have shown it has done to avoid civil litigation or criminal prosecution. But this may be a long way from ideal or even 'good enough' practice. An example is the mindless approach to child protection that assumes that if all staff working in a service have undergone checks through the Criminal Records Bureau (in Britain) then enough has been done to ensure the safety of the children who use the service. This is an example of where relying on a legal procedure may paradoxically make managers complacent and less vigilant in supervising direct care staff. (CRB checks are not foolproof. They can only identify people with a history of convictions, not potential offenders or previous offenders who have not been convicted.)

Research evidence indicates that ethical practice of workers within an organization is not so much related to the quality of its written protocols and procedures but to its *social ethos* (Dubnick 2003; Avshalom and Rachman-Moore 2004). This ethos influences individual workers but is also created in the first place by individual workers themselves—by their individual moral attitudes expressed in practice. The protocols and procedures should flow out of, or at least resonate with, the attitudes of the workers, not be externally imposed upon them. Where this happens it is natural for staff to adopt a critical (though not cavalier) attitude to written guidelines, applying their own personal morality and professionalism as external modulators. Staff *ownership* of and involvement in developing local policies is therefore vital for good practice.

It should be remembered that guidelines for good practice do not exist in a vacuum. They are developed in the service of a higher order goal. Sometimes they will need to be modified in the light of higher order strategic plans. These plans aim at long-term horizon goals and form the backdrop to local immediate practice. The excellent British National Service Frameworks (part of the NHS Plan for improving public health) are examples of the setting within which local practice protocols and procedures are devised. The sorts of strategic developmental considerations dealt with by these frameworks provide another critical perspective on local practice protocols and procedures.

5.2.11 Practice principle 11. Give greatest weight to the agency, distinctive identity, and freedom of the patient when considering what is in his or her interests

This is a simple rule that essentially boils down to the idea that the starting assumption for ABI rehabilitation is that the principle of beneficence is equivalent to the principle of autonomy, and where 'patient autonomy' and 'duty of care' appear to conflict the principle of autonomy should take precedence unless there are very strong arguments against it. It means seeing rehabilitation from the perspective of the patient and driving rehabilitation from the perspective of the patient. It therefore means prioritizing the activities listed under Practice principle 3, treating them as central rather than peripheral to treatment.

This of course involves risk. Minimizing and managing risk is therefore vital if this principle is to be enacted. (It is rarely possible or even desirable to eliminate risk altogether.) One important component of risk management concerns the patient's competence to make decisions.

5.2.12 Practice principle 12. Assess and maximize the patient's competence/capacity to make specific decisions and communicate his or her wishes

I use the term 'competence' to refer generally to the individual's ability to make decisions based on her values and wishes in the light of an accurate appraisal of her situation. The term 'capacity' has essentially the same meaning but tends to be used in a more technical legal sense (see for instance The Mental Capacity Act 2005).

It is important that assessment of competence is not seen as a low frequency activity that only comes into play when legal questions of capacity arise. It is good clinical practice to consider systematically the competence of patients with ABI to assist the team in making informed decisions about the need for paternalistic action. Assessment is not carried out for its own sake but with a view to managing, and if possible improving, the patient's situation. Assessment of competence is a basic component of risk assessment and management but, more importantly, it should also contribute to the promotion of the patient's agency (Practice principle 3). Promoting agency is not just about supporting the enactment of the patient's decisions but about establishing conditions for the patient to make decisions effectively. Effective decision making is not the same as making a 'good' decision. The role of the clinical team is to ensure that the *process* of decision making is optimized, not to determine the *content* of the decision that is reached.

This view is consistent with the basic principles of Mental Capacity Act (2005), one of which is the requirement to take all practicable steps to help a person make his own decisions, and another the right of a capable person to make unwise decisions. The right to make unwise decisions arises from English case law:

> An individual should not be regarded as lacking capacity merely because he makes a decision which would not be made by someone of ordinary prudence. Although the law requires an individual to be capable of understanding the nature and effect of a transaction or decision, it does not require him to behave in 'such a manner as to deserve approbation from the prudent, the wise, or the good'
>
> Bird v. Luckie (1850; 8 Hare 301)

Another feature of the law concerning capacity is that capacity refers to specific decisions, it is not a general condition of the individual. For instance one could be deemed capable of marriage but not capable of handling one's own finances. In clinical practice this is also an important consideration. The question to be asked is 'Is the patient competent to take *this* decision?' Again, in law, people are presumed to have capacity unless incapacity has been clearly demonstrated. The same assumption should apply in the clinical assessment of competence. Finally, competence may change over time. Indeed it is very likely to do so in the case of those recovering from ABI. So it should be regularly reviewed.

Several factors need to be considered in the assessment of competence to make a decision. These include the nature of the decision, the patient's cognitive status, her mental state, her comprehension of the situation in question (both in general terms and in relation to her part in it), her cultural background, and her relationship to others who may exert undue influence. Ideally cognitive status should be assessed by a neuropsychologist and mental state by a neuropsychiatrist. (Some people with ABI sometimes have significant pre-existing or acquired mental health difficulties. Even if their cognitive abilities are relatively good their competence may be called into question because of the presence of delusions or hallucinations.) Other information should be gathered from members of the clinical team, family, and carers.

For competence to be demonstrated the person should, *under optimal conditions*, be able to:

- have sufficient information to be able to reach a simple functional (rather than complex technical) understanding of his situation
- understand the range of possible courses of action
- relate this to his wishes and values
- identify a desired outcome
- make a decision that brings together the information he holds, his wishes and values, and is directed towards achieving the intended outcome, and maintain this decision over a specified time period
- communicate his decision effectively.

Some further reading that provides detailed guidance on assessing competence and capacity is provided at the end of this chapter.

The setting up of optimal conditions is important. A person with memory impairment may not be able to recall all the information relevant to reaching a decision unless provided with information in written or tape-recorded form. A person with verbal comprehension problems may need information to be presented pictorially. A person who does not speak English will need a translator. Any symptoms of severe mental illness will need to be successfully controlled by appropriate medical or psychological treatment. A person with executive problems may need support in linking together the information at his disposal with his wishes and values in order to generate an intended outcome. A person with verbal expression problems or motor problems that affect speech may need help in communicating his wishes. A person who tires easily should make decisions when he is refreshed, and information may need to be presented in bite size chunks. The process of reaching a decision may need to be gone through several times.

One area in which the assessment of competence is important is that of consent to treatment. This issue is hugely significant in ABI rehabilitation. Treatment often begins when the patient is unconscious and therefore clearly not competent to give informed consent. In the early stages of recovery the patient is often irritable, confused, and disorientated. He may resist any intervention that involves touching or handling. This resistance may involve verbal and physical aggression. Early on in rehabilitation a pattern may be established of staff inflicting procedures on a patient who resists aggressively.

Unlearning this pattern of mutual fear and aggression can be one of the challenges of post-acute rehabilitation. The clinical team and the patient under its care have to construct a means of negotiating small routine activities of treatment and care, together with strategic decisions about courses of treatment, length of stay in hospital, place of discharge, etc. The degree of formality required in obtaining informed consent for treatment will realistically vary. Formal explicit consent should be obtained for procedures that carry risk of irreversible detrimental changes, more informal tacit consent is appropriate for routine daily care-giving. But the principle of the patient giving her informed consent to all actions that affect her should form a strong basis of all clinical practice.

Gaining informed consent to treatment involves the following components:

- Assessing competence to make a decision about the proposed treatment
- Establishing optimal conditions for competence
- Optimizing the voluntary nature of the decision. This means ensuring that the patient is not under coercion, for instance fearing she will be discharged from the service if she does not comply with a recommended course of action
- Presenting the evidence on which the decision should be based (for instance degree of pain involved, likelihood of success in achieving a desired outcome, risk of making things worse, *alternative possibilities*)
- Recommending a course of action
- Checking that the evidence presented and the recommended course of action have been understood (for instance, by asking the patient to summarize the pros and cons of different options)
- Asking the patient for her decision and her authorization of action.

The recommendation of a particular course of action should be given by a person with expertise and experience, so that the patient has reasonable grounds to place trust in her judgement. Under some circumstances a patient may prefer to defer to the expertise of a professional whom she trusts. (Recently, when I was in great pain I was presented with three alternative options, together with their various pros and cons, by a doctor. He was clearly a caring and competent professional so I told him I was in too much pain to make a decision and asked him to recommend one. I then consented.) This is acceptable, and often the most appropriate course of action if the decision is technically complex or needs to be taken quickly. Nevertheless, the process of providing information in a comprehensible form, so that the basis of the professional recommendation is clear, should not be bypassed.

The professional should also be *disinterested*. For instance, it is clearly unethical for a doctor in the pay of a particular pharmaceutical company to recommend a drug produced by that company as if on clinical grounds alone.

Despite best efforts, some patients will remain incompetent to take some decisions, and their wishes may have to be overruled. Or competent patients may make antisocial decisions and action to safeguard the interests of others may have to be taken. There are also grey areas, for instance when a patient whose competence is 'borderline' plans a course of action that puts him at considerable physical risk. This is where the 'very strong arguments' against giving priority to the agency of the patient (Practice principle 3) come into play and paternalistic decisions can be justified. Clear written justification for paternalistic decisions should always be given, and the fallout from paternalistic decisions should always be managed.

Treating a person against his will constitutes assault under the law. Because people with ABI can be said to have a mental disorder under the terms of the Mental Health Act 1983/2006 ('an impairment in or disturbance of the mind resulting from any disability or disorder of the mind or brain') or impaired judgement under the terms of the Mental Health (Care and Treatment) (Scotland) Act 2003, it is possible to treat them against their will if due process has been followed. Detaining a person against her will may be more difficult because the Human Rights Act 2002 is highly protective of the 'right to liberty' (Article 5), although some allowance is made for 'mental disorder'. In practice many people with ABI and other disabling conditions are essentially detained against their will without the necessity of the institution's invoking the law. The situation arises through various combinations of their being unable to move independently in order to escape, having insufficient cognitive skills to find the exit, or being unable to communicate their wishes. This is a morally disquieting situation.

5.2.13 Practice principle 13. Acknowledge and manage distress caused by necessary paternalistic action

It is obvious that paternalistic decisions will cause distress to the patient concerned. It is perhaps less obvious that the staff who take and enact a paternalistic decision also experience some discomfort, perhaps even significant distress. One way of dealing with distress is denial of inner conflict, insisting that there is not an issue, and that the decision taken was unequivocally correct—'We couldn't have done anything else' when in fact there were several alternatives. While this may help to a degree, it does not allow any sort of empathy with the patient who feels a decision was unequivocally wrong.

Empathy with the patient is especially important when paternalistic action is taken. Explicit respectful acknowledgement of the patient's views and feelings should accompany action that has been taken in opposition to them. The fact that the patient's autonomy has been compromised should be openly admitted and regretted, not rationalized away.

It should be emphasized that paternalistic decisions are often reversible. Detaining a person in a residential setting against his will may be the correct course of action now, but discharge home may be the longer-term goal. While this may be obvious to the staff team, it should be communicated clearly to the patient. If a decision is to be reviewed, the patient should be told the expected date of review. This gives hope.

Sometimes a paternalistic decision in one area can be mitigated by compromising with the patient's wishes in another less vital area. The patient may have to remain in a residential setting permanently because her beloved home, shared with her beloved dog, is no longer safe given her acquired disabilities. But can a supported setting that accepts pets, or at least where pets can visit, be found for her?

5.2.14 Practice principle 14. Do not impose your personal or professional values on the patient

Our personal values can be so much a part of our assumptive world that they feel like non-negotiable facts rather than opinions: 'abortion is murder,' 'people have a right to know the truth whatever the cost', 'anyone who believes in God is deluding himself', 'people should do things because they want to—not to earn a bribe' and so on. As we take on professional roles we also take on professional values: 'cognitive therapy is demonstrably superior to psychodynamic counselling in all circumstances,' 'physiotherapy is the backbone of rehabilitation', 'rehabilitation is about increasing independence', 'alternative therapies are unproven and worthless', and so on.

We might like our patients and colleagues to behave in conformity with our values, but the reality is that they often depart from them. Even if we were able to force them to behave in a way that we thought was right we would have a hollow victory, for behaviour that is coerced is not moral behaviour at all. So we need to find a way of being alongside people whose behaviour from time to time violates our moral sense or professional values.

Where this sort of mismatch arises and causes us discomfort it may help to try and see how the other person has arrived at his point of view by gentle questioning. Understanding where the other person is coming from is not the same as condoning his position, but may also identify more common ground than was at first apparent. This applies both to professional interactions (for instance a discussion between an occupational therapist and a neuropsychologist about the value of certain tests of cognitive function), and to clinical situations (for instance the discussion between a nurse and her patient about a proposed termination). These sorts of *open* minded discussion can also result in one or both of the parties *changing* their minds, because what has been going on is not unlike humanistic counselling.

Being prepared to change our minds is important, because we are asking our patients to be equally open minded. They may need to reconsider all their initial ideas about future career, life partner, and place of residence. As noted on p. 84 they may also change priorities and even their values. They will certainly be reconsidering their assumptions about the kind of place the universe is. The patient in transition is not an empty vessel into which the therapist can pour her value-driven ideas. He is someone who requires the support of an open-minded fellow traveller. This requires the ability to step outside one's own world view for a while, something that is easier to do if one's world view is secure and respected by others (see Practice principles 18 and 19).

5.2.15 Practice principle 15. Clarify the nature and extent of your duty of care

This is something that requires a good deal of personal reflection and team discussion. There is no universal answer to the question of what duty of care entails, and it should be determined in the light of local circumstances. This process involves both 'thinking outside the box' (Practice principle 4) and its opposite, drawing boundaries.

A minimal duty of care would be the preservation of life, but many would want to include some notion of optimizing 'quality of life' (with all its problems of definition). Some may take a *laissez faire* attitude, understanding the promotion of a patient's autonomy to mean just letting him do what he likes with few or no constraints. Others would understand it to involve a process of gradually reducing support. Others would see it as encouraging the patient along paths that fitted with their own view of the good life, for instance actively educating the patient to promote health-related behaviours or actively encouraging creative endeavours.

There will also be a range of opinions on the management of risk. Does duty of care entail protection from physical harm and minimizing risks at all costs? If not what is an acceptable level of risk? Most people with ABI do not learn to walk again without falling. Sometimes they may sustain significant injuries. What is a 'safe discharge'? It is the nature of ABI to render people more vulnerable to physical accident and injury, and emotional and financial exploitation. Rehabilitation staff, patients, and families have to learn to live with significant risks—*to recalibrate notions of safety* (McGrath and King 2004). Conflict in this area, fuelled by professional values of the sort discussed under Practice principle 14, is one major contributor to conflict in clinical decision making. Explicit discussion of these issues with all parties involved is the basis for resolving it.

5. 2.16 **Practice principle 16. Use evidence-based interventions**

It is relatively easy to carry out research on therapeutic interventions delivered in a uniform manner to a homogenous group of patients. Multidisciplinary brain injury rehabilitation is much more difficult to evaluate because the variability of the patients requires individualized programmes—there are no standard interventions, only standard principles. Thus the whole may be more than the sum of its parts. For instance, it is now well established that specialist stroke rehabilitation units achieve better outcomes for patients with stroke than general hospital wards (e.g. Indredavik *et al.* 1999), but identifying the 'active components' of the package offered continues to present a challenge. Selecting an appropriate outcome measure from the plethora available can be daunting. (See Wade 1992 and Fleminger and Powell 1999 for helpful reviews.)

Randomized controlled trials (RCT), double blind where possible, and involving large numbers of patients, is the method of choice in medicine. Rehabilitation procedures can be fitted into this model with some ingenuity (for instance in 2003 one issue of the journal *Clinical Rehabilitation* included eight studies described as RCTs), though often some artificiality. Nevertheless the requirements of this method may not be suitable or practicable.

Alternative methods should also be considered, especially methods that can be incorporated into clinical practice without too much additional effort. Sophisticated single case studies, using appropriate statistics, can provide robust evidence that a particular intervention is at least an option worthy of rational consideration (Wilson 1987). This can be built on with a series of single cases that strengthen the argument in favour of the intervention (see for instance Wilson *et al.* 2001).

Qualitative methods can also contribute to knowledge, most usefully by enriching rather spare statistical data, by suggesting avenues worthy of further exploration, and by posing challenges to received wisdom by enabling research participants rather than investigators to set the agenda (See for instance Hammell 2003).

Different professions have different attitudes to research methods (see Practice principle 14). For instance doctors tend to prefer quantitative methods, nurses tend to prefer qualitative methods. Sometimes debates about methodology can become very political. Sadly, because of the editorial policy of research journals the two streams of research tend to inhabit separate worlds. More constructive dialogue between these worlds would be welcome and would do better justice to the clinical data.

There also needs to be better dialogue between professionals and patients and their families in this area. On the whole patients and families have little knowledge of or interest in research methodology. They don't want to know that 50% of people who had this treatment in a published RCT demonstrated a quantifiable improvement. They want to know if the treatment will make a clinically significant difference to *this* patient *here* and *now*. In making a decision about this they are likely to be guided by a combination of desperation and anecdote—'It helped a lady down our road who had something like this and we are prepared to try anything.' This sort of thinking is often seen as uninformed and superstitious—greeted with a wry smile or exasperated eye-rolling by professionals. But it is really just a different approach to ethics and epistemology: 'To do right by the patient one must try anything' and 'There is good reason to believe that a treatment is effective if it worked for an identifiable person.' Until this different approach is recognized and respected as such there is little hope of effective negotiation of an agreed approach to treatment. There will be no communication between cultures.

5.2.17 Practice principle 17. Systematically monitor the degree to which your therapeutic objectives have been achieved

Monitoring the achievement of therapeutic objectives, either for an individual patient or across the service as a whole, is in the spirit of using evidence-based interventions. It is essentially the incorporation of a research attitude into routine clinical practice, but is often distinguished from research and described as 'clinical audit'. In fact the demarcation line between research and audit is blurred. For instance the practice of goal attainment scaling (GAS) appears to straddle the two. (For a review of GAS in the context of ABI rehabilitation see Malec 1999.) In addition, if the process of auditing outcome imposes significant burdens on the patient it may require a formal consent procedure and systematic ethical scrutiny in much the same way as a research project (Wade 2005).

Therapeutic objectives (proximal goals) refer to future desired states. They are not action plans (McMillan and Sparkes 1999). In these terms, 'For Mr X to dress himself independently on five occasions next week' is an objective, but 'For Mr X to participate in dressing practice' is an action plan—the means by which the objective may be achieved. Notice that the first of these examples is centred on the patient, but the second is centred on professional practice.

As a general rule, it is desirable for therapeutic objectives to be SMART:

- specific
- measurable
- achievable
- relevant
- timed.

However, sticking rigidly to these criteria can inhibit the setting of objectives that are not easily measurable or timed, for instance those referring to relationships or psychological processes. An improvement in the relationship of a couple cannot be prescriptively set to occur 3 weeks later, in the way that independence in showering can. Nevertheless, objectives that refer to relationships and psychological states should be given as much prominence as goals relating to physical independence. A degree of vagueness in goals referring to these domains is acceptable, but efforts should be made to express them at least partly in terms that can be measured (for instance, for the couple to spend time alone together over a weekend without having a major argument).

The relevance of the objectives to actual concerns expressed by the patient should be included in any audit. It is possible for teams to be on the one hand very good at collecting information from the patient, on the other hand very focused at setting objectives, but not to have brought these things together at all.

Counts of objectives achieved are important, but qualitative information can be just as useful, for example examining instances of failures to achieve objectives and recording the reasons. These reasons may include: over- or underestimation of the patient's potential by the team; lack of resources (equipment, housing, etc.); poor professional practice; developments of unforeseen physical complications (epilepsy, infections, etc.); or changes in social circumstance (break up of marriage, loss of job, etc.).

Monitoring the rate of approach to and achievement of therapy objectives is only worthwhile to the extent that the information gathered has a direct impact on clinical practice. It should be used, not filed away.

5.2.18 Practice principle 18. Aim for coherence between your professional practice and your sense of who you are

This is simply to pursue personal and moral integrity and to avoid 'splitting.' Being guided by different principles in different areas of life is inefficient, effortful, and disorientating. It also means that moral responsibility rests with the roles we occupy and not with us as persons (Bauman 1993, p. 19).

So, it is helpful for clinicians to reflect on their world views, philosophy, or religious beliefs and to connect these with the sorts of things that are required of them in the work setting. Many people do not have a full blown world view, philosophy, or religion, but do have a sense of the sort of person they would like to be. That is they think in terms of virtues—to be kind, honest, open-minded, etc. Making connections between the virtues to which they aspire and their day to day behaviour in the work-place builds a sense of being a whole person. This in its turn builds confidence and, paradoxically, enables the ability to step confidently away from cherished virtues and values in order to enter the perspective of others.

Regular appraisals by peers or line managers are routine parts of professional life in many settings. These appraisals could be enhanced by including morality within their scope. For instance questions such as, 'Which parts of my job express my core values and personality?', 'Which parts of my job make me feel uncomfortable because they clash with my values and personality?', 'How might these issues be addressed?' could be included in the process.

5.2.19 Practice principle 19. Be explicit about your personal values if relevant to the situation

This follows on from practice principle 18. Reflecting on one's values involves making them explicit to oneself. Sometimes values only become explicit when they are violated. The violation may call up inexplicably strong feelings—'That patient was ignored. She was not given a voice!—I am outraged!' is suggestive of a value system that holds the rights of the weak and powerless in high regard.

At times these values may not only be made explicit to oneself but may also need to be communicated to others. This is not to impose one's values on another (and indiscriminate self-disclosure should be discouraged), but to make clear where one stands on certain issues, and to give the values their due by articulating them in a more public setting. Because it is never possible completely to enter the perspective of another, it is sometimes helpful to be explicit about the position one is relinquishing in order to attempt to draw alongside them. For instance, it is probably better practice for a clinician who holds no religious beliefs to make this clear to a patient whose religious beliefs are so precious that they are driving his attitude to rehabilitation. 'I do not share your belief that God will heal you miraculously, but I respect it and am trying hard to understand it' is a better attitude than superficial collusion with or dismissal of the patient's beliefs, or pretending to be 'value-free'. Again, a clinician who holds strong views on sexual morality is entitled to request respect for her views and sensibilities from a patient who freely discusses his serial sexual conquests during unrelated therapeutic activities.

This reminds the patient with a tendency to egocentricity that other people have feelings and views; it is a kind of realistic feedback. Where the patient can see her therapist as a moral person, where she too is required to take on moral responsibility (commensurate with her abilities and position in the power hierarchy), this can itself be a humanizing process.

In my own practice I have found it necessary to explain to patients who hold racist views that I do not want to hear them expressed during a session devoted to neuropsychological assessment. But the expression of such views may be a necessary and relevant part of other activities, for instance when exploring why tensions have arisen between two patients of different ethnic origin.

Being explicit about one's values is easiest in a setting where the right to hold values is respected by others. A healthy system encourages the free expression and exploration of staff values, and makes connections between these and clinical situations. One arguable advantage of team working is that if a staff member has a conscientious objection to participating in a specific activity with a patient another team member may be willing to take it on.

5.2.20 Practical principle 20. Make clinical supervision that includes discussion of ethical aspects of practice an absolute priority

It is often difficult to move the discussion in clinical supervision sessions from service management issues on to issues of clinical practice. Including ethical issues in clinical supervision sessions presents even more of a challenge, but their discussion should be a key ingredient rather than an optional extra (Cutliffe *et al.* 1998; Nyland and Lindholm 1999).

Clinical supervisors should provide a supportive and safe space in which the supervisee can explore his feelings in order to reflect on ethical issues (Practice principle 5). Sometimes the supervisor and supervisee may agree to work on some structured objectives in this area. (For an example see Sliwa *et al.* 2002.) The framework for discussion is likely to include published practice standards and guidelines for the profession concerned. Nevertheless the ethical discourse needs to get around and under these to the principles that led to their formulation (Practice principle 10). Often the function of supervision is for the wise and experienced supervisor to 'hold' the discomfort that goes with having made a difficult decision, or to give professional permission not to treat or to cease treatment.

Sometimes it is useful to call in a third party or an outsider with different expertise to advise or facilitate discussion. This is most cost-effective when it takes place as part of group supervision. The third party might be an ethicist or lawyer, or psychological therapist. The approach of cognitive behaviour therapists may be a particularly useful tool in supervision (Bennett-Levy 2006) because it is particularly useful at exploring the link between feelings and core beliefs.

Peer supervision can be highly effective, either in groups (Walsh *et al.* 2003) or through an individual 'critical friend.' Interdisciplinary teams can offer valuable peer supervision focusing on interdisciplinary issues, with each profession bringing a different perspective (Tarvydas and Shaw 1996).

5.3 Conclusions

In this chapter I have presented 20 principles for good and ethical ABI practice, and I have tried to demonstrate that, despite superficial conflict between some of them, they can in fact be reconciled with each other to a degree. But only to a degree. There are still tensions. Similarly, there will always be healthy tensions as well as unhealthy conflict within interdisciplinary teams and between these teams and the people they try to serve. This is simply because 'we' is not the plural of 'I' (Bauman 1993, p. 48).

In the next short chapter I set out a heuristic for making and enacting ethical decisions based on the principles set out above. The heuristic acknowledges that ethical decisions are required when situations are difficult, ambiguous, and evoke conflict. In Chapter 7 this heuristic is applied in a series of worked examples.

Suggestions for further reading

Collicutt McGrath J (2007). Post acute rehabilitation following traumatic brain injury. In A Tyerman and N King, eds. *Psychological approaches to rehabilitation after traumatic brain injury*. Blackwell, Oxford (in press).

British Medical Association (1995). *Advance statements about medical treatment*. British Medical Association, London.

British Society of Rehabilitation Medicine (2002). Clinical governance in rehabilitation medicine: the state of the art in 2002. *Clinical Rehabilitation* **16**, Supplement 1.

Department of Health (2001). *Good practice in consent implementation guide: consent to examination or treatment*. Department of Health, London.

Department of Health (2003a). *Confidentiality: NHS code of practice*. Department of Health, London.

Department of Health (2003b). *What to do if you're worried a child is being abused*. Circular 2003/007. Department of Health, London.

Department of Health and Home Office (2000). *No secrets: guidance on developing and implementing multi-agency policies and procedures to protect vulnerable adults from abuse*. Department of Health, London.

Grisso T (1986). *Evaluating competencies: functional assessments and instruments*. Plenum Press, New York.

Fleminger S and Powell J (1999). Evaluation of outcomes in brain injury rehabilitation. *Neuropsychological Rehabilitation* **9** (3–4) (Special issue).

Hannell K (2003). *Qualitative research in evidenced based rehabilitation: informing practice through qualitative research*. Churchill Livingstone, London.

Kitwood T (1997). *Dementia reconsidered—the person comes first*. Open University Press, Buckingham.

Lush D (2001). Understanding and assessing capacity. In R Wood and T McMillan, eds. *Neurobehavioural disability and social handicap following traumatic brain injury*. Psychology Press, Hove, East Sussex.

Morgan A (2000). *What is narrative therapy?* Dulwich Centre, London.

Lavigna G (2000). *Alternatives to punishment*. Irvington, New York.

Wong J, Clare I, Gunn M and Holland A (1999). Capacity to make health care decisions: its importance in clinical practice. *Psychological Medicine* **29**, 437–446.

References

Adams N (1996). Positive outcomes in families following traumatic brain injury. *Australian and New Zealand Journal of Family Therapy* **17**, 75–84.

Alexander T (1987). *John Dewey's theory of art, experience and nature: the horizons of feeling*. State University of New York Press, Albany NY.

Avshalom M and Rachman-Moore D (2004). The methods used to implement as ethical code of conduct and employee attitudes. *Journal of Business Ethics* **54**, 223–242.

Baltes P and Staudinger U (2000). Wisdom: a metaheuristic (pragmatic) to orchestrate mind and virtue towards excellence. *American Psychologist* **55**, 122–136.

Banja J (1994). Ethics, outcomes and reimbursement. *Rehabilitation Management* **7**, 61–62.

Bauman Z (1993). *Postmodern ethics*. Blackwell, Oxford.

Collicutt McGrath J and Linley PA (2006). Post-traumatic growth in acquired brain injury: a preliminary small scale study. *Brain Injury* **20**, 767–773.

Cutcliffe J, Epling M, Cassedy P, McGregor J, Plant N and Butterworth T (1998). Ethical dilemmas in clinical supervision 2: need for guidelines. *British Journal of Nursing* **7**, 978–982.

Daisley A (2002). *Adjustment of children to parental brain injury*. DClinPsy dissertation, University of Newcastle.

Dubnick M (2003). Accountability and ethics: reconsidering the relationships. *International Journal of Organizational Theory and Behavior* **6**, 405–441.

Department of Health (2003). *Confidentiality: NHS code of practice*. Department of Health, London.

Dewey J (1922/2002). *Human nature and conduct*. Dover, Mineola NY.

Elliott T and Kurylo (2000). Hope over acquired disability: lessons of a young woman's triumph. In C Snyder, ed. *Handbook of hope: theory, measures, and application*, pp. 373–386. Academic Press, San Diego CA.

Gleick J (1988). *Chaos: Making a new science*. Penguin, London.

Hart T and Evans J (2006). Self-regulation and goal theories in brain injury rehabilitation. *Journal of Head Trauma Rehabilitation* **21**, 142–155.

Hope A and Butler G (1995). *Manage your mind*. Oxford, Oxford University Press.

Hooker K (1999). Possible selves in adulthood. In T Hess and F Blanchard-Fields, eds. *Social Cognition and Aging*, pp. 97–122. Academic Press, San Diego.

Indredavik B, Bakke R, Slordahl S, Rosketh R and Haheim L (1999). Stroke unit treatment: ten year follow-up. *Stroke* **30**, 1524–1527.

Linley PA (2004). Positive adaptation to trauma: wisdom as both process and outcome. *Journal of Traumatic Stress* **16**, 601–610.

Malec J (1999). Goal attainment scaling in rehabilitation. *Neuropsychological Rehabilitation* **9**, 253–275.

McGrath J (2004). Beyond restoration to transformation: positive outcomes in the rehabilitation of acquired brain injury. *Clinical Rehabilitation* **18**, 767–775.

McGrath J and Adams L (1999). Patient-centred goal planning: A systemic psychological therapy? *Topics in Stroke Rehabilitation* **6**, 43–50.

McGrath J and Davis A (1992). Rehabilitation: Where are we going and how do we get there? *Clinical Rehabilitation* **6**, 255–235.

McGrath J and King N (2004). Acquired brain injury. In J Bennett-Levy, G Butler, M Fennell, A Hackmann, M Mueller and D Westbrook, eds. *The Oxford guide to behavioural experiments in cognitive therapy*, pp. 337–339. Oxford University Press, Oxford.

McMillan T and Sparkes C (1999). Goal planning and neurorehabilitation: the Wolfson Neurorehabilitation Centre approach. *Neuropsychological Rehabilitation* **9**, 225–230.

Nylund L and Lindholm L (1999). The importance of ethics in the clinical supervision of nursing students. *Nursing Ethics* **6**, 278–286.

Rothwell N, Lavigna G and Willis, T (1999). A non-aversive rehabilitation approach for people with severe behavioural problems resulting from brain injury. *Brain Injury* **13**, 521–533.

Sargent R, Webster G, White S, Salzman T and McGrath J (2000). Enriching the environment of patients undergoing long term rehabilitation through group discussion of the news. *Journal of Cognitive Rehabilitation* **18**, 20–23.

Seligman M (2002). Positive psychology, positive prevention, and positive therapy. In C Snyder and S Lopez, eds. *Handbook of positive psychology*, pp. 3–9. Oxford University Press, New York.

Siegert R, McPherson K and Taylor W (2004). Toward a cognitive-affective model of goal setting in rehabilitation: is self-regulation theory a key step? *Disability and Rehabilitation* **26**, 1175–1183.

Silwa J, McPeak L, Gittler M, Bodenheimer C, King J and Bowen J (2002). Clinical ethics in rehabilitation medicine: core objectives and algorithm for resident education. *American Journal of Physical Medicine and Rehabilitation* **81**, 708–717.

Snyder C (1994). *The psychology of hope: you can get there from here.* Free Press, New York.

Snyder C (1995). Conceptualizing, measuring, and nurturing hope. *Journal of Counselling and Development* **73**, 335–360.

Snyder C, Sympson S, Ybasco F, Borders T, Babyak M and Higgins R (1996). Development and validation of the State Hope Scale. *Journal of Personality and Social Psychology* **70**, 321–335.

Swiercinsky D (2002). Ethical issues in neuropsychological rehabilitation. In S Bush and M Drexler, eds. *Ethical issues in clinical neuropsychology*, pp. 135–163. Lisse, Swets and Zeitlinger.

Tarvydas V and Shaw L (1996). Interdisciplinary team member perceptions of ethical issues in traumatic brain injury rehabilitation. *Neurorehabilitation* **6**, 97–111.

Wade D (1992). *Measurement in neurological rehabilitation.* Oxford University Press, Oxford.

Wade D (1999). Goal planning in stroke rehabilitation: How? *Topics in Stroke Rehabilitation* **6**, 16–36.

Wade D (2005). Ethics, audit and research: all shades of grey. *British Medical Journal* **330**, 468–471.

Walsh K, Nicholson J, Keough C, Pridham R, Kramer M and Jeffrey J (2003). Development of a group model of clinical supervision to meet the needs of a community mental health nursing team. *International Journal of Nursing Practice* **9**, 33–39.

Ward A and Brown M (2004). The good lives model and conceptual issues in offender rehabilitation. *Crime and the Law* **10**, 243–257.

Webster G and Daisley A (2005). A family resource pack for working with children affected by familial acquired brain injury, *Clinical Psychology* **46**, 26–29.

Wilson B (1987). Single case experimental design in neuropsychological rehabilitation. *Journal of Clinical and Experimental Neuropsychology* **9**, 527–544.

Wilson B, Emslie H, Quirk K and Evans J (2001). Reducing everyday memory and planning problems by means of a paging system: a randomized controlled crossover study. *Journal of Neurology, Neurosurgery and Psychiatry* **70**, 477–482.

Chapter 6

A heuristic for managing ethical dilemmas

In this short chapter I present a simple checklist to help manage the sorts of ethical dilemmas that arise in acquired brain injury rehabilitation. The checklist is summarized in Figure 6.1. While it is basically a list of consecutive actions, there are some feedback loops. These indicate that decisions and actions need constant monitoring in relation to both their immediate consequences and the moral principles that generated them in the first place (see discussion on pp. 67 and 71–72).

This heuristic can be applied to the single practitioner, to multidisciplinary teams, or to interdisciplinary teams. However, it is clear that the application of the heuristic becomes more complicated if more people are involved, and if a team is organized on democratic rather than autocratic principles.

Each stage in the process will now be briefly explained.

6.1 Identify the situation as an ethical dilemma

> ... one can recognize the moral self by its uncertainty whether all that should have been done, has been.
>
> Bauman (1993, p. 12)

Be alert to feelings of disquiet in yourself, or expressed by others in words, or worried or uncertain facial expressions. A simple feeling of 'This can't be right?' is sufficient to identify an ethical dilemma. Try and articulate what it is in the situation that doesn't feel right and help others to do the same.

6.2 List all interested parties

To start with, cast your net reasonably wide. Your feelings of disquiet may relate to an interested party that has until now been forgotten (ranging from an ex-partner to the general public). But you will need to cast the net wider still, and be prepared to come across new interested parties. Use the information you have gained about the patient's family relationships, social networks, and job responsibilities to help you (see p. 84). Having cast the net

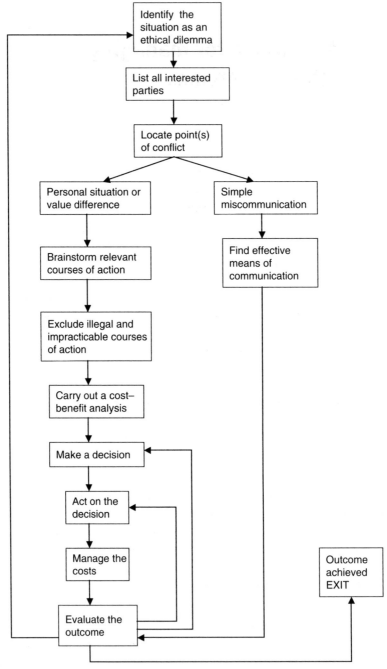

Fig. 6.1 A heuristic for ethical practice

wide, focus down on those people who are really relevant to the current dilemma.

6.3 **Locate point(s) of conflict**

There are several possible points of conflict, some of which are listed below:

- within yourself—between one principle or value and another (e.g. beneficence versus autonomy, your religious beliefs versus your professional aspirations)
- within the professional team—either because of professional differences or personal value differences
- within the patient—between past and present values and goals, or between different aspects of current needs and goals exacerbated by personal fragmentation (e.g. the desire to be pain-free and the desire to walk independently)
- between the patient and her family
- between the team and the patient
- between the team and the patient's family
- between family members
- between family and friends
- between society and the patient
- between the patient and other patients
- any combination of the above!

6.4 **Understand the conflict**

Generally conflict arises as a result of three possible issues, often occurring in combination. Identifying these leads to understanding the situation, and is the basis for its management.

6.4.1 **Miscommunication**

Sometimes conflict arises from simple miscommunication. One or all parties may be ignorant of all the facts. The facts may have been explained by one party but the other party was not able to receive them. In the case of acquired brain injury this is obviously an issue when the patient has significant cognitive impairment, including a specific unawareness of her symptoms (anasognosia). As in the case of capacity (see p. 99) the onus is on the professional to communicate with the patient in a way that ensures both the passing on of relevant facts, and the expression of the patient's wishes and feelings in regard to these. It may then become clear that the conflict was apparent rather than real.

6.4.2 **Personal situation differences—'wheel a mile in my shoes'**

However, there may also be emotional factors that prevent a party from receiving the relevant facts. These factors can influence families and friends as much as (and sometimes more than) they influence the patient himself. It is natural for human beings to protect themselves against the onslaught of potentially devastating information. We do not wish to hear that nothing more can be done, that paying more money or trying an alternative therapist will make no difference, that the prognosis is disappointing, that certain abilities have been irreparably lost, or certain relationships irretrievably lost. The facts may not have been received because the person may not be ready to accept them—may be in denial.

It can be hard for professional teams to empathize with this, to see things from the perspective of the patient and family (see p. 105). The team may want a quick decision from a patient or family member who is just not in an emotional position to make the decision because the massive losses wrought by the brain injury are only just beginning to be processed. Mindful of throughput targets, the team may want to move forward with what will be in the patient's best interests—for instance, purchasing a powered wheelchair for permanent use outdoors, and have little sense what a symbol of defeat and smashed hopes this may be for a patient who had seen a manual wheelchair as an unwanted but necessary temporary aid on the way to independent walking.

There is no short cut to being able to see a particular issue from the patient's perspective. Spending time talking with her and really listening to her is the only way. Identified team members who have special training and proven skills in listening should be called upon here (see Paterson and Scott-Findlay 2002 for a helpful discussion). The patient's perspective may be questionable or even frankly delusional, but it must be fully understood if the situation is to be managed.

6.4.3 **Value differences**

Conflict often arises because of personal and or professional value differences, or because of cultural differences. Cultural differences in attitudes to illness, rehabilitation, and medicine can be very marked and cause a good deal of conflict (see Helman 2001 for a useful review of cultural issues in healthcare). Where a patient comes from a culture that is not well understood by the team then the team may need some inculcation in order to deal effectively with him. Translators or community representatives may have helpful insights to offer here. Networks of healthcare professionals of a wide range of ethnic and national origin can also be a useful resource. Sometimes professionals make too little allowance for cultural difference. Sometimes they make too much allowance:

> There is some evidence to suggest that one of the consequences of an exclusive focus on "culture" in work with black children and families, is [that] it leaves black and ethnic minority children in potentially dangerous situations, because the assessment has failed to address a child's fundamental care and protection needs (Ratna Dutt, director Race Equality Unit, quoted in The Victoria Klimbié Enquiry 2003).

Cultural differences may be more obvious when the patient is a member of an ethnic minority. But there is also a good deal of subcultural variation, especially regarding religion, within the numerically dominant white population, which should also receive attention in seeking to understand conflict.

6.5 Brainstorm all theoretical courses of action

Think of as many potential courses of action *relevant to the ethical dilemma* as possible, taking any personal situational or value differences into account. Be sure to include a 'Do nothing' option. You are unlikely to be overwhelmed with large numbers of ideas—one of the features of ethical dilemmas can be a type of 'idea paralysis.'

6.6 Exclude illegal and impracticable courses of action

Some proposed courses of action will be impracticable because of limited material, financial, or human resources. Others will be clearly illegal. It is simplest to discard these first, and then the relative merits of the remaining actions can be considered.

In Britain a range of legislation is relevant to the management of people with acquired brain injury. Some of this has already been referred to at earlier points in this book. The main legislation to bear in mind is:

- The Mental Capacity Act 2005
- The Mental Health Act 1983/2006 or The Mental Health (Care and Treatment) (Scotland) Act 2003

(There is some overlap between these. Together, they cover competence to make decisions, including consent to treatment, set out the conditions under which a person can be detained and treated against his will, and set out the process for establishing guardianship to secure his best interests.)

- The Children Act 1989 (This is relevant when the interests of children are at stake, especially if there is concern about 'significant harm' to a child.)
- The Human Rights Act 2002 (This is particularly relevant to issues of personal autonomy, for instance the expectation that confidentiality to be respected.)

- The European Convention on Human Rights 1950, 1952, 1963, 1966 (This protects the right to liberty. For instance, where physical restraint is used it should be proportionate, and used only to protect a person from harm.)
- The Health and Safety at Work Act 1974
- The Freedom of Information Act 2000
- The Data Protection Act 1998 (Under this act patients have a right to see their NHS medical records.)
- The Health and Social Care Act 2001 (This is particularly relevant to issues of negligence, for instance in community care settings. Negligence is also covered by the Mental Capacity Act.)
- The Sexual Offences Act 2003 (Sections 34–37 are concerned with protection of persons with a mental disorder from sexual exploitation. Sections 38–44 of this act refer to relationships between care workers and those in their care.)
- The Carers and Disabled Children Act 2000 (This may be relevant to young people acting as carers.)
- Road Traffic Act 1988 and the Driver and Vehicle Licensing Agency (DVLA)'s Medical Rules for Drivers (*www.dvla.gov.uk*)

If there is a concern that a course of action being seriously contemplated may fall foul of the law, then legal advice from an expert should be sought. However, ethical dilemmas tend to arise in situations that have uncertain legal implications. Legal advice may help rule out some courses of action, or draw practitioners' attention to statutory duties of which they had previously been ignorant, *but it will not solve the ethical dilemma.* (And of course some legal actions may be immoral, and some illegal actions moral.)

6.7 **Carry out a cost–benefit analysis**

This is the central part of the heuristic. Consider each remaining proposed course of action, including 'Do nothing' in turn. For each:

1. Specify the *patient's attitude to the intended course of action.*
2. Specify the *intended outcome* (benefits to the patient).
3. Specify the *patient's attitude to the intended outcome.*
4. Estimate the *likelihood of a achieving the intended outcome.* This will be easiest to do, and the likelihood optimized, if the course of action is one that has been tried by others in a similar situation and found to be effective. Clearly, where a recognized clinical treatment is involved consideration of its evidence base is vital.
5. Specify any possible unintended and unwanted outcomes of the action (*risks*), and if possible estimate their likelihood.

6. Estimate the *patient's competence* to decide to undertake this course of action (essentially capacity to consent).

7. Evaluate the *benefits of the intended outcome* according to the criteria set out under Practice principle 3 in terms of whether it will promote the agency, distinctive identity, and freedom of the patient. How likely is outcome X will preserve or enhance B's free and independent movement and action? If B does not wish the course of action to be undertaken, then by its nature it will compromise her agency.

8. Evaluate the *costs of the intended outcome* to other aspects of the patient's interests. How likely is outcome X to impact negatively on A's physical safety, financial security, emotional well-being, mental health?

9. Carry out a similar evaluation for the *other parties* you have identified as interested.

Table 6.1 gives a suggested proforma for each intended course of action. Tables 6.2 and 6.3 give a very simple worked example for a dilemma facing a physiotherapist who is planning treatment of a woman who has multiple severe disabilities resulting from a large cerebral haemorrhage. Even in this simple example it can be seen that some consideration needs to be given to weighing the costs and benefits of the two alternatives—'serial casting of ankle' versus 'do nothing'. There are arguments on both sides.

Table 6.1

	Benefits in terms of agency	Costs in terms of wellbeing
Proposed action		
Patient's attitude to action		
Intended outcome (benefits to patient)		
Patient's attitude to outcome		
Likelihood of achieving intended outcome		
Risks of proposed action		
Competence of patient to decide to undertake action		
Patient		
Interested party 1		
Interested party 2		
Interested party 3		

Table 6.2

Proposed action	Serial casting of ankle	
Patient's attitude to action	Negative—when attempted she screams	
Intended outcome (benefits to patient)	Increased range of movement, possibility of achieving independent standing, assisted walking (a few steps), improved health, access to a wider range of final placements	
Patient's attitude to outcome	Unknown because of major communication and cognitive problems.	
Likelihood of achieving intended outcome	50% chance of achieving increased range of movement. Realistically the chances of achieving independent standing are very low because of her cognitive problems	
Risks of proposed action	The procedure is painful. She may become very distressed and cease to cooperate in other areas of her treatment.	
Competence of patient to decide to undertake action	She is not competent to make a decision regarding this treatment	
	Benefits in terms of agency	Costs in terms of wellbeing
Patient	Some possible long term benefits (but unlikely to be achieved).	Pain, distress, less tolerant of being handled.
Interested party physiotherapist	Therapist is able to carry out treatment of choice aimed at increasing independence of patient.	Therapist feels distressed and guilty at inflicting an unpleasant procedure on her patient

Table 6.3

Proposed action	Do nothing	
Patient's attitude to action	Positive—seems to like to be left alone	
Intended outcome (benefits to patient)	Psychological wellbeing improved (left in peace)	
Patient's attitude to outcome	Unknown because of major communication problems	
Likelihood of achieving intended outcome	Likely—she seems more at ease when not handled intensively, but accurate estimate of her mental state is not possible	
Risks of proposed action	The ankle deformity may get somewhat worse, she may become less tolerant of being handled	
Competence of patient to decide to undertake action	She is not competent to make a decision regarding her treatment	
	Benefits in terms of agency	Costs in terms of wellbeing
Patient	Her apparent wish not to be handled in this way has been respected	Her foot deformity *might* get somewhat worse, she *may* become less tolerant of being handled
Interested party Physiotherapist	?	Therapist feels unprofessional at having not administered treatment

6.8 **Make a decision**

In this instance the 'do nothing' option appears preferable because the costs of the alternative to the patient are clear and its benefits are less likely to be realized. (It could also be argued that the first option should only be considered if the woman is sectioned under the Mental Health Act due to a 'disorder of the brain', because it would otherwise constitute an assault under law. But, as discussed on p. 101, this is a grey area. Under the Mental Incapacity Act 'acts in connection with care or treatment' for a person who is not capable of giving consent are permissible. But is serial casting such an 'act'?)

The final decision made will depend on a combination of factors that include the estimated magnitude of the benefits and costs together with the likelihood that these will be realized. Some costs are so great as to be clearly unacceptable (for instance, significant risk of physical injury to a child) and will rule out a course of action. Otherwise, the decision is likely to be difficult. Nevertheless, laying out the issues systematically, as on the proforma given here, should make it less difficult, aid communication at the time, and provide a record as to why a particular decision was reached.

It is important that responsibility for the decision, whether individual or team, is made explicit and recorded.

6.9 **Act on the decision**

Once a decision has been taken it should be enacted. Where a team is involved named individuals should be assigned to the task(s) specified. This will often include someone designated to keep the patient and family informed of the decision. If the course of action is complicated it may be broken down into stages, with the objective (preferably SMART) of each stage specified.

6.10 **Manage the costs**

All courses of action have associated costs. These costs should be anticipated and managed. In the example given here the potential costs of carrying out serial casting are for the patient increased pain and distress, and decreased tolerance of being handled in other care situations. The physiotherapist is also likely to experience distress. So, a pain management strategy, and positive handling experiences (e.g. massage) could be planned for the patient, together with an opportunity for the physiotherapist to debrief or share the treatment with a colleague.

The potential costs of doing nothing are a worsening of the foot deformity, and a decreased tolerance of being handled due to less frequent handling. The therapist is likely to feel frustrated and unprofessional at withholding treatment.

Again, positive handling experiences should be explored for the patient, and the physiotherapist should make use of supervision to discuss the professional issues raised in deciding not to treat a 'treatable' condition.

6.11 **Evaluate the outcome**

Formal evaluation at a set time after the decision has been reached should be built into the process. The timing of this will depend on the nature of the clinical situation. The questions that need to be asked are:

- Was the course of action decided upon initiated?
- How far has it progressed?
- To what extent has the intended outcome been achieved?
- To what extent have the anticipated risks been realized?
- Has the patient's situation (including competence) changed?
- Have other unforeseen events occurred?

In the example given here, if the serial casting of the ankle had been decided upon then it would be necessary to check that this was being carried out, to check the improved range of movement and functional mobility of the patient, to check the patient's expressions of distress and reaction to handling in other situations, to check that the patient's cognitive and communication abilities have not dramatically improved, and to respond to the unforeseen (for instance, the arrival from abroad of a relative who strenuously objects to the treatment plan).

This evaluation should then lead either to ensuring the plan of action really is being carried out, or continuing with it because it is on course, or terminating it because the desired outcome has been achieved, or reviewing the decision because the costs now appear to outweigh the benefits, or initiating the whole process again because a new ethical dilemma has emerged (in this case the interests of an additional interested party into the equation).

It should be noted that evaluating the outcome will from time to time mean biting the bullet and admitting that the decision made was not a good decision. Living with the consequences of a decision is part of ethical practice. This can be emotionally difficult, but the process described above diverts the focus from guilt and blame on to how to make things better.

6.12 **Conclusions**

As in all rehabilitation, the ethical decision making process outlined in this chapter is recursive. Information gathering leads to a decision, which is followed by action, which is followed by more information gathering, further decision, action modification, and so on. The example given is highly simplified, yet illustrates a number of the complexities involved in the process. In the next chapter we will encounter a series of more complicated cases, each presented as a worked example, and still somewhat simplified. In none of these cases is there a single 'right' way to proceed. The aim is to think as clearly as possible about the issues, to find a systematic way to approach them, and to maintain a patient-centred ethos based on compassion, wisdom, and hope.

References

Bauman Z (1993). *Postmodern ethics*. Blackwell, Oxford.

Helman C (2001). *Culture, health and illness: an introduction for mental health professionals*. Arnold, London.

Paterson B and Scott-Findlay S (2002). Critical issues in interviewing people with traumatic brain injury. *Qualitative Health Research* **12**, 399–409.

Working with diversity. The Victoria Klimbié Enquiry: Report of an enquiry by Lord Laming presented to the Secretary of State for the Health and the Secretary of State for the home Department by Command of Her Majesty, January 2003, Part Five, paragraphs 16.1–16.9.

Chapter 7

Case studies

In this final chapter there are 18 case studies presented as worked examples. Each case study takes the form of a brief scenario followed by a list of issues that it raises. For cases 1–6 the groundwork for decision making set out in Figure 6.1 (see p. 114) is worked through, and completed proformas for alternative courses of action are presented. But no decisions are reached. This is left to the reader(s), as is thinking through the process of enacting the decision, managing the costs, and evaluating the outcome.

Cases 7–12 are worked through less fully because the proformas are not completed. These and all subsequent steps are left to the reader(s).

Cases 13–18 are simply presented together with a list of relevant issues.

These cases are to be worked through essentially from scratch by the reader(s).

The case studies can be worked on by individuals, but they may be most useful as the basis of a group discussion, workshop, or teaching session.

7.1 Case 1: Andy and his family want to travel abroad to try an expensive treatment that has no scientific basis

7.1.1 Scenario

Andy has sustained a severe head injury as the result of a fall, and it has been complicated by a large intracerebral haemorrhage in the right frontal hemisphere. Andy's left arm is paralysed and his left leg is weak. He is extremely passive and his thinking is rather concrete and rigid. His cognitive stamina is much reduced. He appears to have poor insight into his situation. Before his injury Andy was very active, if not driven, and took a major role in the family business, which is very successful.

Andy has undergone nearly a year of intensive of rehabilitation as an in-patient and day patient. His physical progress has been slower than expected, and the rehabilitation team attribute this to his acquired cognitive problems and poor initiative. The professional team members are all agreed that further dramatic improvement is unlikely. In particular, further recovery of arm function is likely to be limited. They believe that it would be in Andy's best interests to return home to be with his wife and young children, to reintegrate into family life, and to work on functional tasks of daily living with support from community services.

However, Andy's father and brother have decided to take Andy abroad for several months to a private clinic offering a treatment of unproven benefit aimed at improving function in his left arm. The treatment will be intensive, and no other rehabilitation will be offered. Andy and his wife have agreed to this plan.

Andy's father and brother want the rehabilitation team to rubber stamp their decision, and to co-operate if required in providing clinical information for the private clinic. But the team members are worried that this inappropriate and expensive treatment will only delay the process of coming to terms with the reality of Andy's situation, that he will forget the functional compensatory skills he has learnt in his rehabilitation, and that he will be further marginalized from family life. They are also uncomfortable at being asked to collude with a questionable clinical approach.

7.1.2 Some issues raised

- The family's difficulty in coming to terms with the situation
- The foregrounding of Andy's father and brother and lower visibility of Andy, his wife, and children
- Andy's competence to agree to the proposed course of action
- The use of evidence in clinical decision making
- The need to maintain a co-operative relationship between Andy, his family, and the rehabilitation team
- The feelings evoked by the implication that because more can be done somewhere else not enough has been done by this rehabilitation service

7.1.3 Groundwork

- Interested parties: Andy, Andy's wife, Andy's children, Andy's father, Andy's brother, the rehabilitation team

- Point of conflict: Understanding and acceptance of situation, attitude to empirical evidence. This could be because of simple lack of knowledge and miscommunication and it is therefore worthwhile putting significant effort into communicating the prognosis and the evidence for it more effectively to all interested parties. However, it appears that there is more to this situation than simple miscommunication, and differences in perspective and situation will remain to be explored further.

- Personal situation perspective: Andy and his family are not emotionally ready to accept the guarded prognosis, and they are particularly reluctant to face the issue of cognitive losses. They want to try everything possible to improve the degree of physical recovery. It is also difficult for Andy to see things from an alternative perspective because of his cognitive problems. Andy is highly influenced by the male members of his family.

- Value perspective: Andy and his family are wealthy entrepreneurs, and their wealth has been accumulated only in the last two generations. Their experience is that apparently insuperable hardship and difficulty can be overcome through effort, and that money can solve most problems.

- Possible relevant courses of action:
  1. Agree to family's request
  2. Refuse family's request
  3. Take legal action to protect Andy from his family.

- Impracticable or illegal course of action: The legal basis for action plan 3 would be very shaky. Despite his cognitive losses it would be difficult to argue that Andy lacks capacity to agree to his family's plan. In addition, the proposed ineffective treatment is not known to have any specific unwanted side-effects. Therefore, only action plans 1 and 2 need to be considered.

7.1.4 Cost–benefit analysis

Both Tables 7.1 and 7.2 identify costs that will need to be managed if the particular action plan is followed, in these cases the identification and possibly provision of sources of emotional support for the family or rehabilitation team.

The proformas deal with the alternatives facing the team when presented with what is essentially a *faîte accompli* by the family. However, it would also

Table 7.1

Proposed action	Support family in their decision to send Andy to a private clinic and to cooperate with the process by sharing clinical information
Patient's attitude to action	Not bothered either way
Intended outcome (benefits to patient)	The private clinic would be working from good information. Keeping family on side would mean that other clinical recommendations might be more readily accepted. It would also be easier to resume treatment or pick up pieces if the private clinic doesn't work out.
Patient's attitude to outcome	Andy would probably like to maintain a good relationship with this rehabilitation team.
Likelihood of achieving intended outcome	Good, especially if view of the team is assertively stated, and a distinction drawn between personal support (yes) and action endorsement (no).
Risks of proposed action	Family might learn that they can 'dictate terms' to rehabilitation team.
Competence of patient to decide to undertake action	Andy is not central to this interchange which is between team and family. He has been assessed as competent to consent to the treatment plan favoured by his family.

	Benefits in terms of agency	Costs in terms of wellbeing
Patient Andy	The course of action to which he has agreed has been supported	Coming to terms with situation may be put back
Andy's father and brother	Their chosen plan has been supported and their means of coping respected	Coming to terms with situation may be put back
Andy's wife	Negligible	None
Andy's children	Negligible	None
Rehabilitation team members	Very little. A high degree of value compromise	Frustration, sense of being disempowered and under-valued

Table 7.2

Proposed action	Refuse to support family in their decision to send Andy to a private clinic, not cooperating with the process by sharing clinical information
Patient's attitude to action	Not bothered either way
Intended outcome (benefits to patient)	The family might rethink its decision and fall in line with the view of the rehabilitation team, Andy would be spared exposure to an ineffective treatment and could spend time with the family
Patient's attitude to outcome	On his own, Andy *might* be persuaded that discharge home is preferable
Likelihood of achieving intended outcome	Zero. Andy's father and brother insist on sending him to the private clinic. Andy will follow their advice.
Risks of proposed action	Andy and his family might become alienated from the rehabilitation team. The private clinic would be working from hearsay information. The team might not be able to help in the future because of relationship breakdown with the family.
Competence of patient to decide to undertake action	Andy is not central to this interchange which is between team and family. He has been assessed as competent to consent to the treatment plan favoured by his family.

	Benefits in terms of agency	Costs in terms of wellbeing
Patient Andy	None	Distress at family anger or falling out with rehabilitation team
Andy's father and brother	None	Negligible
Andy's wife	Negligible	Distress at family anger or falling out with rehabilitation team
Andy's children	Negligible	Negligible
Rehabilitation team members	A sense of being true to professional values	Distress at family anger and losing relationship with Andy

Table 7.3

Proposed action	To take Andy to a private clinic abroad for intensive treatment of his left arm impairment	
Patient's attitude to action	Positive, but he tends to be heavily influenced by the male members of his family	
Intended outcome (benefits to patient)	Improved arm function, with a knock on effect on general function	
Patient's attitude to outcome	Positive	
Likelihood of achieving intended outcome	Low. There is no evidence that the treatment is effective.	
Risks of proposed action	Loss of existing rehabilitation gains, marginalization in family circle, distancing from wife and children, children, delay of coming to terms with situation, diversion from more important rehabilitation activities	
Competence of patient to decide to undertake action	Patient is on balance competent but he doesn't appreciate the wider ramifications of his decision	
	Benefits in terms of agency	Costs in terms of wellbeing
Patient Andy	Uncertain: Is this really Andy's 'own' decision? If arm function *could* be improved this would be beneficial.	Marginalization, loneliness, loss of rehabilitation gains, delay in coming to terms etc.
Andy's father and brother	Clearly beneficial *if* treatment works. If not, at least they can say they did all they could.	Coming to terms with situation may be put back
Andy's wife	None. Has anyone asked *her* what she really wants?	Loss of relationship with Andy. Marginalisation from decision making
Andy's children	Ditto	Potentially damaging separation from father

be possible to use them to help the family review its own decision. An idea of how this might be done is presented in Table 7.3.

7.2 **Case 2: Barbara wants to die**

7.2.1 **Scenario**

Barbara has sustained a brainstem stroke. She is unable to move her limbs or to speak, but she can communicate using eye pointing and a simple communication aid. Her swallow reflex is not secure and is fed through a percutaneous endoscopically guided gastrostomy (PEG). Barbara has been in hospital for a year and physical improvement has been very limited. Her cognitive skills are good, and she has been able to negotiate a programme of care where she is reasonably well in control of what happens. Barbara is single and has one sister living. She was previously a teacher and held strong views on the rights of very sick and disabled people to choose when and how to end their lives.

From time to time over the last year Barbara has expressed a desire to be 'put out of my misery'. More recently she has articulated this wish more clearly and has formally asked the clinical team to assist her in her wish. Her sister does not agree with Barbara's views but feels that her wishes should be respected. The members of the rehabilitation team are deeply and passionately divided in their views on the issue.

7.2.2 **Some issues raised**

- Is Barbara depressed?
- Could her 'quality of life' be better?
- Can dying ever be in a person's best interests?
- Other people in Barbara's position seem to cope and even to love life.
- If Barbara wasn't so disabled she could end her own life, but then her reason for wanting to end her life would not be so pressing.
- Is Barbara being selfish to expect this help from others?

7.2.3 **Groundwork**

- *Interested parties.* Barbara, Barbara's sister, members of the rehabilitation team, groups in society with a wider agenda on the 'right to die'
- Point of conflict: For some members of the rehabilitation team there is a conflict between the principle of autonomy and the principle of benefi-cence, for some there is an additional conflict with religious beliefs about the sanctity of life, for some members of the rehabilitation team and for Barbara there is no such conflict. For Barbara's sister there is a conflict between her desire to keep her sister with her, her own beliefs, and the

desire to respect her sister's wishes. It is very important in this case to make sure that good information is made available to all concerned. In particular Barbara must have good information about her impairments and her prognosis. She must also have good information about what her future life is going to be like as a lived experience. That is, she must be allowed to experience hope that things can better. Barbara may be depressed, and her mood should be formally assessed and, if necessary treated. However, Barbara's pessimistic view may simply be based on negative experiences in hospital and ignorance of what may available to her once discharged into the community. (For instance she may assume that she will always have to live in an institution.) Barbara cannot make an informed decision about her own future life unless she has good information and an opportunity to experience the best possible life given her impairments. Because this may take time to organize, responding to her request can be postponed, at least for a while, though her wishes should be formally acknowledged and recorded. An opportunity to talk with trained 'listeners' will be important. Barbara may then change her mind. But she may not.

- If the request persists then it is likely to come from a stable perspective and to express enduring personal values.
- Possible relevant courses of action:
    1. refuse to expedite Barbara's request in any way
    2. assist Barbara in her suicide
    3. encourage Barbara's sister to assist her in her suicide
    4. support Barbara in becoming sufficiently independent (for instance in accessing the internet) for her to be in touch with people who will help her travel to a country where physician-assisted suicide for people in her situation is tolerated by the law
- Impracticable or illegal courses of action: Action plans 2 and 3 are illegal and can quickly be ruled out. Therefore only action plans 1 and 4 need to be considered (Tables 7.4 and 7.5).

7.2.4 Cost–benefit analysis

This case is highly morally charged and carries with it a significant degree of perceived risk. In cases like this professionals often passively slide into a 'do nothing' option (essentially action plan 1, but without making the costs explicit, or attempting to manage them in any way.) Another common option is 'pass the buck' on to the next link in the chain of rehabilitation and care services. In this way the issue is avoided, but the autonomy of the patient is not respected.

Table 7.4

Proposed action	To refuse to expedite Barbara's request for assisted suicide in any way
Patient's attitude to action	Very negative
Intended outcome (benefits to patient)	Barbara will remain alive. She will have the opportunity to change her mind.
Patient's attitude to outcome	Very negative
Likelihood of achieving intended outcome	Good, especially if combined with careful observation and limitation of Barbara's activities in this direction
Risks of proposed action	Barbara may despair and become depressed
Competence of patient to decide to undertake action	Barbara is completely competent to refuse to comply with this approach, though unable to enact her wish

	Benefits in terms of agency	Costs in terms of wellbeing
Patient Barbara	None—what little she has is deeply is deeply compromised.	Physical life but psychological despair and possible physical deterioration
Barbara's sister	She is unsupported in attempting to respect her sister's wishes, but supported in her own views on the wider issue.	Distress caused by Barbara's despair, and possibly more pressure on her from Barbara to address the issue
Rehabilitation team member who favours principle of assisted suicide	None	Frustration and sadness at Barbara's despair
Rehabilitation team member who objects to principle of assisted suicide	Beneficial. Professional and personal values endorsed	Guilt at ignoring patient's clearly stated wish. Sadness at Barbara's despair
'Political' interest groups	None	None

Table 7.5

Proposed action	Support Barbara in becoming sufficiently independent for her to be in touch with people who will help her achieve her goal within the law	
Patient's attitude to action	Positive, but would prefer a more direct approach to the issue	
Intended outcome (benefits to patient)	Barbara's wishes will be respected and supported. She will be the active director of her fate.	
Patient's attitude to outcome	Positive	
Likelihood of achieving intended outcome	Good, though it is not certain that Barbara will be able to effect all the necessary actions to achieve her goal	
Risks of proposed action	The team could cross the line from rehabilitation aimed at maximising autonomy to active collusion with Barbara's plans, painting her into a corner so that she would lose face if she changes her mind. This is a serious risk that should be carefully monitored and legal advice sought.	
Competence of patient to decide to undertake action	Barbara is completely competent to engage with this approach.	
	Benefits in terms of agency	Costs in terms of wellbeing
Patient Barbara	Highly beneficial because responsibility is handed back to Barbara	If she achieves her goal—loss of life
Barbara's sister	Negligible, but pressure is off her	Sadness and unease at her sister's life choices. Loss of sister.
Rehabilitation team member who favours principle of assisted suicide	Beneficial. Professional and personal values endorsed	Unease at this choice for *this* patient
Rehabilitation team member who objects to principle of assisted suicide	None	Major distress at any suggestion of collusion in a process that may end in assisted suicide

Table 7.5 *(cont.)*

	Benefits in terms of agency	Costs in terms of wellbeing
'Political' interest groups	'Euthanasia' agendas may be advanced if Barbara goes public	'Right to life' agendas may be impeded if Barbara goes public

7.3 Case 3: Chris intends to drive but he is not safe to be on the road

7.3.1 Scenario

Chris has driven for many years, both professionally and for pleasure. He loves cars, and has taken part in cross-country driving events. He has sustained a stroke involving the right cerebral hemisphere. This left him with left visual field loss and left inattention and neglect, which have got less troublesome as his recovery has proceeded. He has poor insight into his cognitive losses. He has made a good physical recovery, lives at home alone, and attends out-patient rehabilitation sessions, travelling by public transport.

Six months after the stroke Chris tells several members of the team that he intends to take his sports car out of the garage and go for a drive. He has been told on several occasions that he must surrender his licence to the DVLA and cannot legally drive until it is returned to him. Unless his visual field loss has shrunk to negligible dimensions the licence will not be returned. But Chris is evasive whenever the subject is mentioned, and the team suspects that he never returned his licence to the DVLA.

7.3.2 Some issues raised

- Chris's right to confidentiality
- The moral obligation of the rehabilitation team to other road users
- The legal obligation of the team
- The team's duty of care in relation to Chris

7.3.3 Groundwork

- Interested parties: Chris, other road users, the police.
- Point of conflict: It is possible that Chris does not fully understand the legal requirement to surrender his licence and the fact that driving without a licence is illegal. This should be carefully explained to him. A formal letter might help to drive the point home. However, he may have such poor insight into his medical condition that he believes that the law does not

apply to him. He may have anasognosia—a belief that he has not had a stroke, or that his stroke has not caused any difficulties that are relevant to driving. If the problem is anosognosia then Chris' competence to make a decision regarding his licence is called into question.

- Personal situation perspective: Driving has been central to Chris' sense of who he is. The prospect of giving it up may be very painful. His procrastination at surrendering his licence may reflect emotional resistance, and his words about taking the car out on the road may be merely bravado. This requires more exploration and, if necessary Chris should be offered

Table 7.6

Proposed action	Do nothing	
Patient's attitude to action	Positive—or has Chris disclosed his intention because he wants the team to take responsibility out of his hands?	
Intended outcome (benefits to patient)	Chris' confidence has been respected. He has been encouraged to take responsibility for his own actions	
Patient's attitude to outcome	Positive—or is Chris 'really' asking for help?	
Likelihood of achieving intended outcome	Good	
Risks of proposed action	Despite appearances Chris may 'really' prefer the team to be more proactive. But this doesn't appear very likely.	
Competence of patient to decide to undertake action	Chris' competence to decide to drive his car is highly suspect.	
	Benefits in terms of agency	Costs in terms of wellbeing
Patient Chris	Clear benefits	Chris could kill or injure himself
Other road users	None—they have not been consulted	Risk of death or injury on road increased
The police	None—they have not been consulted	They are road users too.
Rehabilitation team members	None	They are road users too. Guilt and sense of responsibility for Chris' actions.

Table 7.7

Proposed action	Inform the police	
Patient's attitude to action	Negative	
Intended outcome (benefits to patient)	No benefits in terms of agency and freedom. Perhaps a police warning would help the development of insight.	
Patient's attitude to outcome	Negative	
Likelihood of achieving intended outcome	Moderate	
Risks of proposed action	Chris could become very angry and more fixed in his intention to drive. He might even retaliate by driving when unsupervised without heed to the consequences. The team would have broken his confidence and he might try and take legal action. His likelihood of success would be low, but it would be an unpleasant process for all concerned.	
Competence of patient to decide to undertake action	Chris' competence to decide to drive his car is highly suspect. Formal assessment of capacity is advisable.	
	Benefits in terms of agency	Costs in terms of wellbeing
Patient	None	Possible emergence of behavioural disturbance or other forms of distress— depression
Other road users	Their chances of staying alive, and thus freedom, increased	Increased danger on roads if Chris 'acts out'
Police	Have information on which to act	Negligible
Rehabilitation team members	Have taken responsibility	Guilt at breaking patient's confidence

Table 7.8

Proposed action	Try and get Chris legally detained for residential treatment	
Patient's attitude to action	Negative	
Intended outcome (benefits to patient)	Increased insight into the reality of his situation and hence greater freedom to make informed choices	
Patient's attitude to outcome	Does not see need for this	
Likelihood of achieving intended outcome	Low to moderate. It is not certain that the law would support this action, and problems with insight respond best to specialist programmes which may not be readily available.	
Risks of proposed action	Chris may become angry and refuse to cooperate or develop more challenging behaviour.	
Competence of patient to decide to undertake action	Chris is probably not competent to make a decision regarding residential treatment.	
	Benefits in terms of agency	Costs in terms of wellbeing
Patient Chris	None immediately— possibly some longerterm benefits	Possible emergence of behavioural disturbance or other forms of distress— depression
Other road users	Their chances of staying alive, and thus freedom, increased	None
Police	Negligible	Negligible
Rehabilitation team members	Have taken some responsibility	Unease at participating in detention against the patient's will

emotional support as he goes through the process. But if Chris' intentions are real then the rehabilitation is faced with a number of options.

- Possible relevant courses of action:
  1. do nothing (ignore the situation)
  2. inform the police

3. try and get Chris admitted to hospital under the Mental Capacity or Mental Health Acts so that his insight can be worked on more intensively.

- Impracticable or illegal courses of action: All three options are practicable and (arguably) within the law (Tables 7.6, 7.7, and 7.8).

7.3.4 Cost–benefit analysis

None of these options is particularly attractive or low on risk. The final decision will depend on the relative weight given to the interests of the patient and the interests of wider society.

7.4 Case 4: Doris is so homesick in the rehabilitation unit that she has considered suicide but she will be at physical risk if she is discharged home

7.4.1 Scenario

Doris has a history of heavy drinking. About 6 months ago she sustained a significant head injury as the result of a fall at home when she was under the influence of alcohol. She has made a good physical recovery and, apart from a tendency to forgetfulness, her cognition is relatively good. However, her mood is depressed and is getting worse. She often weeps and constantly asks when she can go home. Doris says that she would consider suicide if she could not return to her home.

Doris' husband left her many years ago, and her only daughter, who used to share her home died in tragic circumstances. Her most important relationships are with her two cats, whom she greatly misses.

The occupational therapist has observed that, although she is frail, Doris is fairly independent and safe in carrying out self-care and domestic activities. But she is concerned that Doris may begin to drink again, and under those circumstances she may fall, or set the terraced house on fire if she falls asleep while smoking.

7.4.2 Some issues raised

- How to manage a fluctuating state
- Is it right to detain someone against her will where the risks are uncertain?
- Protecting the patient from physical harm may amount to inflicting an equal degree of psychological harm
- The rights of other residents in the road
- The clinical judgement of risks and therefore the sense of responsibility rests with a single profession

7.4.3 **Groundwork**

- Interested parties: Doris, Doris' neighbours, the occupational therapist.
- Point of conflict: The occupational therapist is in a conflict situation. She understands the issues around mood, functional independence and safety, duty of care, and paternalism. There are no significant difficulties in communicating with Doris, but the issue may not have been fully and clearly discussed with her precisely because her therapist is paralysed by conflict.

Table 7.9

Proposed action	Transfer Doris to a residential care setting	
Patient's attitude to action	Extremely negative	
Intended outcome (benefits to patient)	Physical safety and opportunity for a good life if the residential setting is chosen sensitively, particularly if pets can be accommodated, and if counselling is available to address long standing loss issues.	
Patient's attitude to outcome	Extremely negative	
Likelihood of achieving intended outcome	Low. Transfer may be effected (though legal position should be confirmed), but residential options are limited, and Doris is unlikely to have a positive attitude to it.	
Risks of proposed action	Doris may become more depressed, attempt or carry out suicide.	
Competence of patient to decide to undertake action	Doris is essentially competent to refuse the transfer.	
	Benefits in terms of agency	Costs in terms of wellbeing
Patient Doris	None	Significant costs in terms of mood. Possible loss of life.
Doris' neighbours	Their houses are less likely to catch fire.	None
Occupational therapist	Questionable	Guilt at having overridden patient's clear wishes

Table 7.10

Proposed action	Discharge Doris home	
Patient's attitude to action	Very positive	
Intended outcome (benefits to patient)	Return to her own cherished environment where she can be independent and resume her relationship with her cats	
Patient's attitude to outcome	Very positive	
Likelihood of achieving intended outcome	Good, especially if a high input care package is in place and if Doris will accept some safety adaptations to her home.	
Risks of proposed action	Doris might injure herself (quite likely) or set her house on fire (less likely).	
Competence of patient to decide to undertake action	Doris is essentially competent to take the decision to return home.	
	Benefits in terms of agency	Costs in terms of wellbeing
Patient Doris	Significant — her wishes are respected and her sense of identity supported	A degree of physical risk, especially if she drinks heavily
Doris' neighbours	None — they haven't been consulted	A possibility (small) that their houses may catch fire
Occupational therapist	Questionable	Guilt at not having acted 'responsibly'. Worry about fire risk.

Help and support from other team members should be provided, and a formal psychiatric evaluation carried out. Nevertheless, the bottom line is that Doris is desperate to go home and her therapist does not feel able to plan a discharge home.

- Personal situation perspective: All Doris' memories are associated with this home, where she brought up her daughter. Her current important relationships are centred on this home. She cannot envisage a care environment in which she would be able to keep cats. Doris is frustrated and bored in the rehabilitation unit, and in fact her in-patient rehabilitation is essentially complete.

She longs for her own space and old lifestyle, so much so that she is experiencing a type of bereavement reaction.

♦ Value perspective: Doris sees alcohol as a positive enhancer of her quality of life, and her way of coping with the bad memories that might otherwise overwhelm her.

♦ Possible relevant courses of action:
  1. discharge Doris to a residential care setting
  2. discharge Doris home
  3. do nothing
  4. transfer Doris to a setting for people with mental health problems

♦ Impracticable and illegal courses of action: Action plan 3 is not an option because there is pressure to clear beds in the unit. Action plan 4 is not practicable because these services are already pressured and Doris does not meet their admission criteria. Therefore only action plans 1 and 2 need to be considered (Tables 7.9 and 7.10).

7.4.4 **Cost–benefit analysis**

This seems to be a no-win situation for the therapist. If she is part of a team it is important that the responsibility for decision making is explicitly shared. If not, she should insist on supervision and support from her managers. It seems natural to respond with sympathy to Doris' request when she is present in the room, but the decision might be different if the small children who live next door were also present.

7.5 **Case 5: Elizabeth wants to care for her children but while she has been in hospital her family have employed a nanny**

7.5.1 **Scenario**

Elizabeth has sustained a stroke involving the left cerebral hemisphere. She was in hospital for 6 months and now attends a rehabilitation unit as a day patient. She has a right-sided weakness and major problems with expressive language. She is able to walk and is learning to carry out some functional tasks with her left hand.

Elizabeth is married and has three children aged 3, 7, and 11. She was previously a full-time homemaker. During her time in hospital her husband and sister decided to employ a live-in nanny. Elizabeth wants to resume her role as primary caregiver of her children, and the rehabilitation team have been supporting her. However, her husband and sister believe that this is an unrealistic goal and wish to retain the nanny on a long-term basis. They will not cooperate

Table 7.11

Proposed action	Continue with rehabilitation aimed at Elizabeth resuming her role as primary caregiver, hoping that the family can be talked around	
Patient's attitude to action	Positive, as far as can be ascertained	
Intended outcome (benefits to patient)	Family will come to some agreed compromise that will allow Elizabeth to take on significant but not necessarily exclusive role in caregiving.	
Patient's attitude to outcome	Positive	
Likelihood of achieving intended outcome	Uncertain	
Risks of proposed action	Avoiding confrontation may weaken Elizabeth's position and allow existing arrangements to be consolidated	
Competence of patient to decide to undertake action	Elizabeth's language difficulties prevent her from understanding the subtleties of this approach	
	Benefits in terms of agency	Costs in terms of wellbeing
Patient Elizabeth	Elizabeth's goals are being addressed *to an extent*	Negligible
Elizabeth's husband	Some—his opinion is respected in negotiations	Negligible
Elizabeth's sister	Ditto	Ditto
Elizabeth's children	If their opinion is sought then there are benefits	Negligible
Rehabilitation team member who prioritises disabled parents' rights	Negligible	Unease that team is being insufficiently proactive
Rehabilitation team member with high child care standards	Negligible	Unease that team is colluding with patient's unrealistic expectations

Table 7.12

Proposed action	Seek legal representation for Elizabeth	
Patient's attitude to action	Positive	
Intended outcome (benefits to patient)	Protection of Elizabeth's rights of access to the children will be and increased chances of her resuming her role as primary caregiver	
Patient's attitude to outcome	Positive	
Likelihood of achieving intended outcome	Uncertain (primary caregiving) to good (rights of access)	
Risks of proposed action	Antagonising family could make Elizabeth's position more difficult. Increased family tension could affect wellbeing of children. Family cooperation with rehabilitation programme could cease.	
Competence of patient to decide to undertake action	Elizabeth's appears capable of understanding the legal position in general terms.	
	Benefits in terms of agency	Costs in terms of wellbeing
Patient Elizabeth	Good—Elizabeth's agency is being supported	Increased family tensions could cause significant distress
Elizabeth's husband	None	He is likely to be distressed, anxious, and possibly angry
Elizabeth's sister	None	Uncertain
Elizabeth's children	If their opinion is formally sought then there are benefits	They could get caught up in family antagonisms
Rehabilitation team member who prioritises disabled parents' rights	Good	Negligible
Rehabilitation team member with high child care standards	Negligible	Unease that team is taking sides inappropriately

Table 7.13

Proposed action	Rethink the rehabilitation plan
Patient's attitude to action	Negative
Intended outcome (benefits to patient)	Elizabeth will not be given false hopes. She can begin to come to terms with the reality of her situation and focus her efforts on things other than motherhood.
Patient's attitude to outcome	Negative
Likelihood of achieving intended outcome	Changing rehabilitation plan is achievable, but Elizabeth may not cooperate.
Risks of proposed action	Elizabeth could become depressed or angry and uncooperative. Continuing minimal contact with her children could cause them distress
Competence of patient to decide to undertake action	Elizabeth is on balance competent to dispute the approach, but she would need significant support in expressing her views.

	Benefits in terms of agency	Costs in terms of wellbeing
Patient Elizabeth	None	Major distress, possible setback to progress in other areas
Elizabeth's husband	Good—his wishes are respected	Little chance of his coming to understand Elizabeth's perspective
Elizabeth's sister	Ditto	Ditto
Elizabeth's children	Uncertain	They could suffer from lack of familiar contact with their mother
Rehabilitation team member who prioritises disabled parents' rights	Poor	Significant distress
Rehabilitation team member with high child care standards	Good	Negligible

with the rehabilitation programme, believing this to be giving Elizabeth false hopes, and that it is not in the interests of the children to receive primary care from a person with significant physical and communication impairment.

The rehabilitation team is split. Some members feel Elizabeth's wishes should be supported at all costs. Others feel that there may be some wisdom in her family's analysis of the situation.

7.5.2 **Some issues raised**

- The interests of children are sometimes in conflict with the interests of parents
- The difference between a disabled person becoming a parent and a parent acquiring a disability
- To what extent can a rehabilitation team 'interfere' with a marriage?
- Does rehabilitation entail being an advocate for the patient?
- Do professionals overidentify with patients of the same sex and similar age and background?

7.5.3 **Groundwork**

- Interested parties: Elizabeth, Elizabeth's husband, Elizabeth's sister, Elizabeth's children, the rehabilitation team members
- Point of conflict: The conflict is between Elizabeth and her husband and sister, between members within the rehabilitation team, and possibly between Elizabeth's interests and that of her children.
- Personal situation difference: Elizabeth expects and wishes to become close to her children again and to resume her role as a mother. It seems that Elizabeth's husband and sister are not fully aware of Elizabeth's perspective. They see Elizabeth primarily as a disabled person. This may be for emotional reasons, and if this is so psychological work with the adults in the family may be desirable, but it may also be resisted. In addition this sort of psychological work is difficult if one of the parties has major communication problems.
- Value difference: Some would argue that the right of a disabled person to be a parent should be paramount. Others would argue that the right of children to be cared for by a person with minimum competence in certain areas is paramount. As far as the rehabilitation team goes it might be helpful to make use of an independent facilitator, for instance a group therapist or ethicist.
- Possible relevant courses of action:
  1. continue with rehabilitation aimed at Elizabeth resuming her role as primary caregiver, hoping that the family can be talked around

2. seek legal representation for Elizabeth to protect her rights of access to the children and further her agenda of resuming her role as primary caregiver

3. re-think the rehabilitation plan, encouraging Elizabeth to accept that she will have a marginal role in her children's care, and focus on alternative rehabilitation goals

◆ Impracticable or illegal courses of action: All three action plans are practicable, though action plan 1 might be difficult to sustain for long. (Tables 7.11, 7.12, and 7.13)

7.5.4 Cost–benefit analysis

These proformas do not do justice to the breadth of Elizabeth's rehabilitation needs because they focus on one question—her relationship with her children. Her relationship with her husband is arguably just as important and is not fully addressed in this discussion. Indeed this is yet another conflict—she may only be able to preserve one relationship at the expense of the other.

7.6 Case 6: Fred needs a prostitute

7.6.1 Scenario

Fred is a single man who comes from another part of the country. Fred was always a loner, but found pleasure and meaning in regular encounters with prostitutes. He sustained a severe head injury as the result of a road traffic accident 9 months ago while driving on business. He also sustained some orthopaedic injuries.

He is not able to walk more than a few steps and uses a wheelchair most of the time. Fred's cognition is reasonable, though his concentration is poor, and he tends to persist with certain favourite themes in conversation. He is thought to be ready for discharge to sheltered accommodation in his home town, but there is some delay in arranging this.

Fred is quite sexually explicit in his conversations with direct care staff and enjoys explicit magazines which he is able to purchase at a local shop. It is not clear whether his preoccupation with sex is a result of the head injury or expresses his frustration at nine months' sexual abstinence.

Fred is very keen to make contact with local prostitutes. He says he is very lonely and depressed and wishes to 'prove his manhood' and reassure himself that he is the same person as before the accident. As he does not know the area he asks the nursing staff to help him organize the contact and transport. Some of the nurses feel very comfortable to help him in this way. Others are deeply offended at the request.

7.6.2 **Some issues raised**

+ Are Fred's requests symptoms of 'disinhibition' that need to be treated?

+ What is the legal position?

+ Would it be acceptable to leave this to the discretion of individual staff members?

+ What is the risk of sexually transmitted disease?

+ Will Fred put ideas into other patients' heads?

+ It is usually nurses who are under most pressure in the rehabilitation of intimate functions. How can they best be supported by the rest of the team?

7.6.3 **Groundwork**

+ Interested parties: Fred, nursing staff (also consider hospital managers, other patients, prostitutes?)

+ Point of conflict: This seems to be a difference in values between Fred and some of the nursing staff.

+ Personal situation perspective: Fred has probably always been someone with limited means of coping, with poor social and relationship skills. He has relied heavily on relationships to which he brings his money rather than himself. The change in circumstances arising from the head injury has completely cut him off from his familiar local environment and his one source of pleasure and meaning. His tolerance of frustration has probably been reduced further through damage to the frontal areas of the brain.

+ Value difference: Some members of the nursing team feel that Fred's autonomy and agency should be supported. If he were not physically disabled and far from home he would use prostitutes anyway. He will do so in the future. So, it is right to support and facilitate his agency in this important area. Other team members feel that what Fred is doing is wrong—it damages both him and the women he uses. Supporting him would not only make them culpable but would bring the whole rehabilitation service into disrepute.

+ Possible relevant courses of action:

  1. facilitate Fred's finding a prostitute and travelling to meet her

  2. ignore Fred's request (do nothing)

  3. refer Fred for specialist treatment aimed at improving his social and relationship skills and managing his preoccupation with sex

+ Impracticable or illegal courses of action: It is possible that action plan 1 is illegal because it could be argued that it amounted to the procurement of sex for a vulnerable adult by people whose duty was to care for that adult (Sexual Offences Act 2003). This is likely to depend on whether Fred is

Table 7.14

Proposed action	Facilitate Fred's finding a prostitute and travelling to meet her
Patient's attitude to action	Positive
Intended outcome (benefits to patient)	Fred's will have achieved his goal, which is aimed at enhancing his sense of identity and self worth.
Patient's attitude to outcome	Positive
Likelihood of achieving intended outcome	Good—this is a habitual coping response which has worked in the past.
Risks of proposed action	It is possibly illegal therefore specialist advice should be sought. Fred may have a humiliating experience. Fred may contract a sexually transmitted health condition.
Competence of patient to decide to undertake action	On balance Fred appears competent to make this decision

	Benefits in terms of agency	Costs in terms of wellbeing
Patient Fred	Good	Other ways of dealing with Fred loneliness and frustration will not be explored. Opportunity for personal growth missed. Some sexual health risk.
Member of nursing team who prioritises patient autonomy	Good	Negligible
Member of nursing team who prioritises sexual morality	None	Significant distress

Table 7.15

Proposed action	Ignore Fred's request
Patient's attitude to action	Negative
Intended outcome (benefits to patient)	Fred may give up and turn his attention to other aspects of his rehabilitation
Patient's attitude to outcome	Uncertain
Likelihood of achieving intended outcome	Possible — but Fred has been very persistent in his requests and tends to get fixed on certain topics.
Risks of proposed action	Fred's loneliness and frustration may develop into depression or aggression. Or he may make sexual advances to other patients or members of staff.
Competence of patient to decide to undertake action	No decision is required of Fred.

	Benefits in terms of agency	Costs in terms of wellbeing
Patient Fred	None	Possible deterioration in mood or behaviour
Member of nursing team who prioritises patient autonomy	None	Frustration and unease at ignoring patient's wishes
Member of nursing team who prioritises sexual morality	Good	Possible unease that the issue has not been addressed directly

judged to have the capacity to decide to have sexual relations with a prostitute. All three action plans will be considered but legal advice should be sought in connection with action plan 1.

7.6.4 Cost–benefit analysis

In this sort of case, where the way forward is unclear, and the patient is not physically able to cause a lot of trouble, the 'do nothing' option is often embraced. An alternative unstated option is 'turning a blind eye'—that is passive collusion rather than active facilitation. In this case Fred might discreetly persuade a visitor to the unit who shares his values to put him in

Table 7.16

Proposed action	Refer Fred for specialist treatment aimed at improving his social and relationship skills and managing his preoccupation with sex	
Patient's attitude to action	Uncertain	
Intended outcome (benefits to patient)	Fred could achieve greater personal freedom if more coping responses and relationship options were open to him.	
Patient's attitude to outcome	Uncertain	
Likelihood of achieving intended outcome	Some progress might be made, though Fred may be too set in his ways (compounded by frontal lobe damage) to change dramatically. Accessing an appropriate service may prove difficult.	
Risks of proposed action	Minimal	
Competence of patient to decide to undertake action	Fred may have difficulty seeing the point of this proposal due to a combination of cognitive impairment, sense of personal identity, and basic values. But it is difficult to argue for formal incapacity in this area	
	Benefits in terms of agency	Costs in terms of wellbeing
Patient Fred	Good—*if Fred agrees to referral*	Few—but some threat to personal identity
Member of nursing team who prioritises patient autonomy	Good—*if Fred agrees to referral*	Some uneasiness at attempt to 'improve' Fred
Member of nursing team who prioritises sexual morality	Good	Negligible

touch with a prostitute and help him organize a taxi. Is turning a blind eye to this behaviour ethically acceptable? Would it be more acceptable if nursing staff try and limit damage by discussing sexual health issues with Fred?

7.7 Case 7: Gordon can only swallow thickened liquids but his family keep feeding him chocolate bars

7.7.1 Scenario

Gordon is a young single man who suffered cerebral hypoxia as the result of an anaesthetic accident. He had never left the family home to live independently. Gordon is very physically dependent and has severe global cognitive impairment. He needs help with all care. His swallow reflex is very unreliable and his speech and language therapist has recommended that he should be fed only thickened liquids and puréed foods. She has provided a written dietary care plan to all staff and to Gordon's parents and older brother.

However, members of the nursing team report that Gordon's family have been feeding him pieces of his favourite chocolate bars when they visit him. When challenged, they respond that Gordon has asked for chocolate and that 'he hates eating slops and has nothing else left to enjoy in life.'

7.7.2 Some issues raised

- Gordon's capacity to make a decision about what he eats
- Is Gordon really asking for chocolate?
- Does Gordon express consistent preferences?
- The family's level of understanding of the risks involved
- The family's difficulty in coming to terms with the situation
- Would the 'old' Gordon have wanted to live this sort of life?
- Local professional practice guidelines or the wider professional literature might help (For a general discussion see Sharp and Bryant 2003.)

7.7.3 Groundwork

- Interested parties: Gordon, Gordon's mother, Gordon's father, Gordon's brother, speech and language therapist (direct care staff, Gordon's friends?).
- Points of conflict: It is possible that Gordon's family do not understand the risks and these should be fully spelt out to them in clear and simple terms. If this does not work, personal situational or value differences need to be identified and addressed. There is also a potential conflict between what Gordon *might* have said had he written an advance directive and what are in Gordon's best interests now.

- Personal situation perspective: It may be that his family cannot accept what has happened, are in denial, and have regressed to a basic form of nurture and care—a personal situational difference. Family counselling might be helpful. It is also possible that Gordon's current state is so distressing to his family that at times they wish he was dead, so the fact that feeding him chocolate increases this risk is not for them an emotionally strong argument against it.

- Value perspective: The family may genuinely think the risks are worth taking in order to improve Gordon's 'quality of life.' This is especially likely if Gordon had ever expressed a view about how he would respond to being severely disabled.

- Possible relevant courses of action:
  1. do nothing
  2. take steps to appoint a guardian for Gordon through the Court of Protection
  3. ban Gordon's family from visiting the unit
  4. offer (PEG) feeding as an alternative to thickened liquids and purées

7.8 Case 8: Harry is locked in his house when his wife goes out shopping

7.8.1 Scenario

Harry sustained a subarachnoid haemorrhage 2 years ago. He lives in the family home with his wife. Harry is forgetful and easily becomes disorientated. He is physically independent but is quite passive, and content to sit in a chair at home for long periods.

It seems possible that Harry's cognitive function is deteriorating, and he is referred by his general practitioner to a clinical psychologist who visits his home to carry out a neuropsychological assessment. She is horrified to discover from care assistants who are present during the examination that Harry is regularly locked in the home by his wife. This is for short periods while she carries out various errands. There are apparently no financial resources or personnel available for continuous supervision at home by care staff. Harry's wife is worried that if she doesn't lock him in he will wander off and get lost or run down by a car. The psychologist challenges Harry's care manager about the situation. He agrees that it 'isn't ideal' but he is concerned that if Harry's wife is confronted she will simply refuse to care for Harry at home any more. He would then have to enter residential care—the one thing he repeatedly says that he dreads. The psychologist, care manager, and general practitioner decide to meet to plan a way forward.

7.8.2 **Some issues raised**

- The legal position—human rights legislation
- Distributive justice—who decides the allocation of resources?
- The needs of carers
- The uncertainty of the risk—is Harry also at risk of setting the house on fire and being unable to escape?
- Pragmatic versus idealistic approaches
- Influencing care conditions in the community is more difficult than in a residential unit

7.8.3 **Groundwork**

- Interested parties: Harry, Harry's wife, community care staff, other service users who require care resources, the clinical psychologist, the care manager, general practitioner.

- Points of conflict: There is conflict between two things that are in Harry's best interests—his freedom to move about in the environment and the opportunity to remain in the home of his choice. There is conflict between the approaches taken by the two professionals involved. There is possible conflict between what is in Harry's best interests and the interests of other service users. There is probable conflict between what is in Harry's best interests and what is in his wife's best interests. However, there is also a lack of good information regarding the risk that Harry will actually wander out into the street if left alone in the house. A formal risk assessment that uses the neuropsychological test results should be carried out.

- Personal situation perspective: Not enough is known about Harry's wife's point of view or any needs for emotional support that she may have. These should be investigated, and it is possible that a sensitive approach may lead to a resolution of the situation.

- Value perspective: Harry's wife apparently prioritizes his safety over his freedom. She seems resigned to the fact that he cannot have both.

- Possible relevant courses of action if the situation cannot be resolved informally:
  1. do nothing
  2. remove Harry to a residential care setting
  3. campaign for sufficient care for Harry to be effectively supervised using human rights legislation if necessary

7.9 Case 9: Ian wants to decorate his hospital room with pictures of topless women

7.9.1 Scenario

Ian is 18 years old and recovering from a severe head injury complicated by multiple orthopaedic injuries as the result of a motorbike accident. His arm movements and speech are ataxic. He has been in hospital and confined to bed in traction for several months. At his request his friends have provided him with magazine pictures, posters, and calendars featuring topless female models and he has pinned many of these up on the walls of his room.

Ian's mother says that his bedroom at home was decorated in this way, and it makes the room feel more like his space. This helps Ian as he is very homesick. Also he is a normal young man and it would be worrying if he did not have normal sexual desires. Some of the nursing staff who have sons of Ian's age are very sympathetic to this point of view, but the younger nurses are uncomfortable when they enter the room to carry out intimate care with Ian.

A new junior doctor is assigned to the ward. She is horrified that such pictures are allowed and refuses to enter the room unless they are removed. She makes the point that the hospital ward is her workspace just as much as it is the patients' home space. She says that the legitimate worries of the junior nurses have been dismissed by their older colleagues as 'inexperience'. Intimate care is being delivered by these women, and a backdrop of topless pinups can only add ambiguity to a situation where boundaries and roles are already fluid.

7.9.2 Some issues raised

- Power dynamics within a professional team
- Sexual harassment in the workplace
- Health and safety at work
- Feminist analyses
- Lack of focus on normal sexuality in rehabilitation
- Territorial issues
- Two-way boundary maintenance in physical care giving
- The personal private domain has become the public domain

7.9.3 Groundwork

- Interested parties: Ian, Ian's family, Ian's friends, older members of the nursing team, younger members of the nursing team, the doctor.

- Point of conflict: This seems to be a value difference with Ian and his family and some rehabilitation professionals on the one hand, and other rehabilitation professionals on the other.

- Personal situational perspective: Ian is at an age when he is very interested in sexual activity and relationships. He was clearly already expressing this interest before his accident, but it did not impinge on public space. It is likely that he was sexually active, or at least that he masturbated regularly. He is now deeply sexually frustrated. He is not in contact with female friends and he is physically incapable of relieving himself. He has little privacy in which to do this. It is also likely that the brain injury has directly affected sexual interest or lack of social inhibition. In addition, Ian is keen to be seen as a 'normal' and fit young person, and the way he wants his room decorated expresses this. There are several ways that these issues could be addressed. There may be other ways to make Ian's room express who he is and feel more like home. Ian may agree to confine his pictures to a folder or other private space, though he would need physical help in accessing them. More attention could be paid to sexual and social relationship issues in Ian's rehabilitation.

- Value difference: For some of the interested parties pictures of topless models are part of the 'real world', harmless—if not beautiful, and a sign of life and health. For others (and this would be particularly true for several religious groupings and those taking a feminist perspective) such pictures are offensive, threatening, and degrading to women.

- Possible relevant courses of action:
  1. insist on removal of pictures from the room
  2. assign only those members of the team who are comfortable in Ian's room to care for him
  3. set up a private space for Ian that is separate from the space in which his physical care takes place, and assist or retrain him in the skill of masturbation.

7.10 Case 10: Joan confides that her partner has hit her

7.10 Scenario

Joan lives at home with her partner. She has no other family. Some years ago she had surgery to remove a benign tumour from the cerebellum. She has poor co-ordination and cannot walk, and uses a wheelchair indoors and out. Her partner is her main carer. Joan thinks and moves slowly, but her cognition is generally reasonable.

Joan has a care manager, but no other community services are involved. She attends out-patient physiotherapy twice a year for review. At one of these reviews she tells the physiotherapist in passing that her partner occasionally hits her. She then begs her not to tell anyone else, especially not the care manager whom she dislikes. Joan says that her partner is very caring on the whole, and only hits her when she 'winds him up'. He hasn't hurt her badly. She definitely does not want to leave him, and she is terrified that he will find out that she has told someone about his actions. She does not think that he would accept support for himself as he is 'a very private person'.

7.10.2 **Some issues raised**

- 'Duty of care' versus 'right to confidentiality' (Human rights legislation places a very strong emphasis on the right to privacy and confidentiality.)
- Sharing confidential information between agencies
- Danger of alerting the perpetrator
- The burden placed on carers
- Joan's capacity—despite the fact that her cognition is 'reasonable' Joan may be in a relationship where she is under undue influence
- Does Joan want to stay in the relationship because there are no attractive alternatives?
- The need for local guidelines and protocols, especially where single practitioners are involved

7.10.3 **Groundwork**

- Interested parties: Joan, Joan's partner, the care manager and social services, the physiotherapist, the general practitioner
- Point of conflict: The physiotherapist faces a conflict between the principle of beneficence and the principle of autonomy.
- Personal situational perspective: Joan may also be in a conflict situation. The relationship is not safe, but the world outside is not safe either for a person with her disabilities who has no family. Her conditional disclosure is perhaps the only thing she can do. She may hope that a magic solution can be found by somebody else, because she certainly can't effect change herself.
- Possible relevant courses of action:
  1. override Joan's stated wishes and alert other responsible care professionals or the police

2. confront Joan's partner and try to persuade the couple to have relationship counselling

3. do nothing other than keep trying to persuade Joan to agree to the wider sharing of the information.

7.11 Case 11: Keith's wife is in another relationship but he doesn't know

7.11.1 Scenario

Keith is an in-patient in a rehabilitation unit recovering from cerebral hypoxia following a cardiac arrest. He has been left with major memory problems. He has also developed a rather facile and childish sense of humour. He is generally impulsive and has a quick temper. He is physically fit and able.

Keith has been married to Sarah for 10 years and they have two children. He has been a devoted husband, and is trying very hard in rehabilitation sessions so that he can return home to his family. The rehabilitation team has been supporting him in this goal, which seems realistic. However, his memory and impulse control are still in the early stages of recovery.

One day Sarah telephones his psychologist to say that she has been in a relationship with another man for 2 years. She says that this was at first just a 'fling', but since Keith's illness this man has been so supportive, and Keith has been so insufferable, that she has decided to end the marriage. Her boyfriend has essentially moved into the family home while Keith has been in hospital.

Sarah feels that the team should know about the situation because it is meaningless to be aiming rehabilitation at return home. But she does not want Keith to know because she thinks that he could not handle the information at this point in his recovery, he might have another heart attack or 'go berserk'. She is certainly not going to tell him—she is afraid of his short temper.

7.11.2 Some issues raised

- Is it always right to tell a person the true state of affairs?
- The timing of disclosure of significant information
- Is lying less of an issue when the person you lied to can't remember what you said?
- The difficulty in rehabilitation planning in uncertain domestic situations

7.11.3 Groundwork

- Interested parties: Keith, Sarah, Keith's children, the rehabilitation team.
- Point of conflict: It may be in Keith's best interests to withhold information from him for a while. But this would involve lying—a conflict between

means and ends. In particular, the rhetoric of the rehabilitation plan would not match its practice: staff would be searching for alternative placements while colluding with the notion of return home.

- Personal situational perspective: Keith is unaware of the situation but his perspective is likely to be that he has a right to know the truth.
- Possible relevant courses of action:
  1. tell Keith the truth
  2. support Sarah in telling Keith the truth
  3. postpone telling Keith the truth, modify the rehabilitation plan, and give him a plausible rationale for the modification
  4. try and persuade Sarah to change her mind.

7.12 Case 12: Laura hardly eats anything

7.12.1 Scenario

Laura has been highly physically dependent for many years as the result of a subarachnoid haemorrhage. She is in residential care. Her speech is very slow and effortful, she has some strange ideas and seems to get stuck in certain themes, but in many respects her cognition appears to be good.

Laura is troubled by numerous symptoms—constipation, headaches, skin rashes, etc. She has read widely, and believes that many of her symptoms are caused by toxins in her diet. She has therefore taken to eating a very restricted diet. Within this she will only accept food that is organic and whose source she can confirm. She will only accept food that has been cooked in spring water.

This regime is very difficult to deliver, and even when catering staff make an effort to do so, Laura is suspicious that they have cut corners. If she feels unwell after a meal she may blame the catering staff for using the wrong ingredients. She sometimes sends meals away untouched because they do not meet her standards. Laura's family and the staff looking after her think her attitude is ridiculous. However, she has a couple of friends who visit regularly and who share her views.

However, it is Laura's body weight that causes most concern to staff. She has always been skinny, and it is proving difficult to maintain her previous weight. They are worried that she may develop bedsores, become weaker, and essentially starve herself to death.

7.12.2 Some issues raised

- When do values become overvalued ideas and when do overvalued ideas become delusions?
- People are usually free to hold odd dietary beliefs and pursue strange dietary practices. Why should a disabled person be any different?

- Does Laura have an eating disorder?
- The carers and catering staff are Laura's proxy arms and legs. Are they entitled to say 'no'?

7.12.3 Groundwork

- Interested parties: Laura, Laura's family, Laura's friends, care staff, catering staff, medical staff.
- Points of conflict: The care staff experience a conflict between the principles of beneficence and autonomy. One way forward might be to have further information on Laura's mental state and cognitive abilities. But assessing mental state in a situation like this is actually a heavily value-laden exercise. There is also a value conflict between staff and Laura's family on one side, and Laura and her friends on the other.
- Personal situational perspective: Laura is completely physically dependent on other people. She has minimal control over her own body. One way that she can maintain strong control is through determining what goes into her body. Food is a compelling bargaining tool because people in caring professions have a strong tendency towards nurture and a horror of physical emaciation. Perhaps this is Laura's way of organizing her own 'death with dignity'?
- Value difference: There is a value difference between the 'mainstream' science of nutrition and perspectives from alternative practitioners.
- Possible relevant courses of action:
  1. initiate PEG feeding against Laura's will using the Mental Health or Mental Capacity Acts
  2. do nothing—let nature take its course
  3. threaten to discharge Laura from this residential setting unless she complies with the normal dietary regime.

7.13 Case 13: Mary won't use contraception

7.13.1 Scenario

Mary is a young woman who sustained a severe head injury as the result of a road traffic accident. There was extensive damage to the frontal lobes. She has made a good physical recovery, and returned home to live with her parents, but has become very disinhibited and impulsive, and has little regard for the consequences of her actions. She goes out a lot and her parents are suspicious that these outings involve casual sex.

Mary previously used the contraceptive pill while in a stable relationship that has now ended, but her mother is sure that she is forgetting to take it.

She persuades Mary to visit her general practitioner to discuss contraception. The general practitioner advises a depot injection. Mary refuses to consider this point blank. She says she hates injections, has no problems remembering to take the pill, and wouldn't care if she got pregnant anyway. She calls the doctor a rude name and storms out of the surgery.

7.13.2 Some issues raised

- Sexual health issues are wider than contraception
- Is Mary a vulnerable adult?
- Mary's right to become a parent
- Who is responsible for Mary?
- There are a lot of people in the community who have not had a head injury and act like Mary. Is Mary's case different?
- What would the 'old' Mary think of her present behaviour?

7.14 Case 14: Neil thinks God will heal him

7.14.1 Scenario

Neil is a university student with a deep Christian faith. He sustained a severe head injury along with multiple orthopaedic injuries as the result of a climbing accident. His memory is very poor and his thinking style has become quite rigid. He has recently been admitted to a rehabilitation unit, and requires intensive and extensive multidisciplinary rehabilitation.

Neil's physiotherapist has become very worried because he is not co-operating in his sessions. When the rehabilitation consultant asks Neil about this he replies that he has had a prophetic word of knowledge that God will heal him, and that no therapy is required. A group of friends from university is also coming to pray and lay hands on Neil. Neil's girlfriend shares his belief, and is arranging for him to attend some faith healing events in another town. This will involve his absence from the unit altogether for a period of 2 weeks.

Neil's parents do not share his faith and are very concerned at the situation. They ask the consultant to 'order' Neil to remain at the unit and to 'compel' him to take an active part in physiotherapy.

7.14.2 Some issues raised

- Cultural difference or mental health issue?
- Neil's capacity to make a choice in this area
- Faith healing event might have a (placebo?) positive effect

- Faith healing event might carry physical and psychological risks
- Religious beliefs of rehabilitation team members are likely to vary

7.15 Case 15: Is it worth trying to do anything more with Olive?

7.15.1 Scenario

Olive sustained a haemorrhagic stroke 5 years ago. She had little in the way of rehabilitation and was transferred straight from an acute hospital ward to a nursing home. She receives good physical care but no stimulation. She weighs 14 stone and is hoisted for all transfers. She seems to be blind and does not speak. Sometimes she smiles.

Olive's children and husband are indignant that she has not had any rehabilitation input. They believe that her potential has not been assessed and that she has been 'left on the scrap heap'. They are successful in organizing a referral to a regional rehabilitation unit.

A speech and language therapist from the unit visits Olive and, on the basis of her examination, is certain that an effective way of communicating with Olive could be found. She also thinks that there is some physical potential and that Olive's vision needs expert assessment. It would be difficult to offer this other than by admission to a specialist multidisciplinary unit. She agrees with the family that Olive has a right to rehabilitation. However, others on the team point out that Olive's heavy care needs would use up resources that could be given to three less dependent patients who have better 'rehabilitation potential.' At the end of the day Olive will probably return to the nursing home, so the benefit in terms of resource use will be negligible. And what if the nursing home fills her bed while she is in the rehabilitation unit? She has all the characteristics of a 'bed blocker.'

7.15.2 Some issues raised

- Distributive justice versus individually based morality
- The criteria of rehabilitation success—absolute level or relative gain?
- The criteria of rehabilitation success—'quality of life' or overall cost saving?
- What about people who don't have family acting as their advocates?

7.16 Case 16: Pauline's 12-year-old son gives her a bath

7.16 Scenario

Pauline shares her home with her 12-year-old son, Joe. Since a stroke affecting her right cerebral hemisphere 3 years ago she has lost the use of her left arm and is only able to walk very short distances. She seems to lack awareness of her environment and is quite disorganized in self and domestic care activities. Pauline receives a care package from social services. As part of this carers are designated to help her with bathing once a week. But Pauline wants to bathe more often, and her carers have discovered that Joe helps her with this, undressing her, manoeuvring her into the bath, and helping with washing and drying.

The carers alert their manager, who is very concerned that a child should be undertaking these sorts of care activities, and astonished that Pauline should think it appropriate. This sort of practice breaches the local guidelines on children as carers.

But when Joe is interviewed by a social worker he says that he particularly enjoys helping his mother in this way. He can remember Pauline doing the same thing for his granddad before he died. Now it's his turn to help his mother in the same way. He feels useful and included, and his mother can have a bath as often as she wants. He is considering a career in nursing. He would be very reluctant to have to give up this activity, and he thinks Pauline would be very upset.

7.16.2 Some issues raised

- Trust and respect for norms and practices within a family
- Does protecting vulnerable children sometimes turn into infantalizing young adults?
- Given her cognitive deficits, is Pauline fit to parent Joe?
- Good practice guidelines don't always have the answer in complex cases
- What is the legal position?

7.17 Case 17: Rashida can't access day rehabilitation services

7.17.1 Scenario

Rashida sustained a left hemisphere stroke 1 year ago. She has been left with right leg and arm weakness. She is almost certainly dysphasic, but this has been very difficult to assess because she only speaks Urdhu.

Rashida lives at home with her extended family. She attends outpatient appointments for medical and physiotherapy review accompanied by her husband and sons who speak for her. She is quite passive during these appointments. It is clear that she is doing less than her physical abilities would predict. She is physically capable of walking, but appears to spend the day sitting watching television at home, and is pushed in a wheelchair on her few trips out to hospital.

Rashida is referred for day rehabilitation. However, she does not attend the centre. When her husband is contacted he says that she doesn't want to come.

7.17.2 Some issues raised

- The disadvantaged position of women in some cultures
- The different attitude to illness and rehabilitation in different cultures
- The importance of keeping the family on side
- Doing nothing could be interpreted as colluding with racist/sexist stereo-typing
- Taking action to change the situation could be interpreted as lack of respect for difference

7.18 Case 18: Should Tom be sedated?

7.18.1 Scenario

Tom is recovering from surgery to remove a pituitary tumour on a neurological ward. He is usually very lethargic, preferring to lie in bed all day, but can get agitated if he is disturbed. His memory is poor and he is disorientated at times. He has no physical impairment, but his muscles have become weak from prolonged activity.

Tom is becoming increasingly aggressive when staff attempt to interact with him. At first he just shouted and screamed. Now he hits out and bites. Nursing staff are scared to enter his room and disturb him. But he needs to be woken up to use the lavatory, and to attend sessions in the hospital physiotherapy and occupational therapy departments.

It would not be possible to institute a behavioural management programme because there is no clinical psychology service for the ward, and insufficient staff to implement any programme with the required consistency. The ward team wonders if the only option is to sedate Tom so that his basic physical care needs can be met.

7.18.2 Some issues raised

- Health and safety at work
- Emotional care of direct care staff
- Sedation is likely to make Tom's lethargy worse
- Sedation is likely to impact negatively on Tom's cognition

- Should Tom be formally sectioned under the Mental Health Act?
- Is lack of appropriate resources a good enough reason for a 'bad' clinical decision?

References

Sharp H and Bryant K (2003). Ethical issues in dysphagia: when patients refuse assessment or treatment. *Seminars in Speech and Language* **24**, 285–299.

Glossary

Activity limitation Difficulty in executing a meaningful task or action.

Advance directive A 'living will' in which the person's views and wishes are set out and which can be invoked if he or she should become mentally incapable of making informed choices about medical treatment, at some future time. The legal status of advance directives is not completely clear.

Affect The general mood state of a person, usually described as positive or negative.

Agnosia The inability to recognise or appreciate the nature of sensory stimuli in a person who has intact sensation and normal alertness.

Alexithymia Difficulty in identifying or describing emotional feelings, which may or may not be underpinned by a loss or impoverishment of affective experience. It is associated with some types of mental health problems but is increasingly recognised as a complication of acquired brain injury.

Alimentary canal The digestive pathway, beginning at the mouth, including the stomach and intestines, and ending at the anus, by which food enters the body and solid wastes are expelled.

Alzheimer's disease Also known as 'dementia of the Alzheimer type' (DAT). A health condition characterised by degeneration of the brain that first appears as memory loss and develops into generalised loss of cognitive function.

Anterograde amnesia The inability to remember events that occur subsequent to a brain injury.

Apraxia The inability to carry out purposeful movements (actions) following damage to the brain, that cannot be accounted for by weakness, inco-ordination, or problems in understanding instructions.

Aristotle A Greek philosopher and early scientist living in the fourth century BCE, author of the **Nicomachaean Ethics**, a work concerned with the search for an 'objective' basis to morality.

Aspiration pneumonia Injury and infection of the lungs caused by the inhalation of food.

Ataxia Muscular inco-ordination and poor balance.

Audit An evaluation of an organization, system, or process in terms of its stated aims and objectives (For instance the length of a service's waiting list.)

Auditory cortex The area of the cerebral cortex in the temporal lobes that is concerned with the perception of sound.

Beneficence The moral principle of doing good.

Brainstem The lowest portion of the brain, continuous with the spinal cord. It includes the pons, medulla oblongata, and midbrain. These are concerned with arousal, basic life functions such as respiration and heart rate, and movement.

Capacity The legally confirmed ability to engage in certain acts. In adults capacity is always presumed. Incapacity has to be demonstrated.

Capgras syndrome A rare delusional belief that a person has been duplicated and is therefore not who he appears to be. It can occur as part of a mental health condition or as a consequence of ABI.

Categorical imperative An absolute, unconditional requirement that holds in all circumstances.

Central nervous system (CNS) The brain and spinal cord.

Cerebellum A distinctive complex structure adjacent to the brainstem concerned with muscular co-ordination and balance.

Cerebral cortex The outer layer of the cerebral hemispheres consisting of 4-6 layers of neurons. It is most phylogenetically recent and is sometimes referred to as 'neocortex'. It is concerned with high level cognitive functions.

Cerebral hemisphere The spherical forebrain is divided into these two large structures with convoluted surfaces, that are essentially mirror images of each other.

Cognitive (behavioural) therapy A branch of psychological therapy that aims to modify unhelpful ways of feeling and acting by focusing on habitual unhelpful ways of thinking. It is generally time limited, highly focused, and collaborative.

Confabulation The experience of false memories, ranging from simple and fleeting to elaborate and fixed, by a person with amnesia.

Confucius A Chinese philosopher with a particular interest in personal and public morality living in the sixth century BCE.

Consolidation The laying down of memory traces in permanent form so that later retrieval is possible.

Contracture A tightening of muscle, tendons, ligaments, or skin that limits normal joint movement. Contractures can occur because of immobility arising from weakness or paralysis or from changes in muscle tone.

Cortical blindness Blindness caused by damage to the visual cortex.

Cortical deafness Deafness caused by damage to the auditory cortex.

Cranial nerves Twelve pairs of nerves arising from the brain stem and spinal cord that carry motor and sensory information between the head and neck and the brain.

Delusion A belief that is opposed to reality and firmly held despite clear evidence that it is not true.

Depot injection A way of administering medication so that is slowly released into the body. This avoids so the need to remember to take regular doses.

Descartes, René (1596-1650). A French mathematician and early rationalist philosopher, with a particular interest in the relationship between the mental and the physical.

Dementia Progressive, permanent, and eventually generalised cognitive impairment associated with progressive, permanent, and widespread changes in brain structure and function.

Distributive justice The principle of fair allocation of benefits and burdens in a society.

Dominant hemisphere/cerebral dominance The cerebral hemisphere that is specialised for language function (usually the left).

Double blind A research design where participants are assigned to various conditions (for instance drug versus placebo) and in which neither the participants nor the investigators know to which condition they have been assigned.

Dysarthria Difficulty in speech production caused by weakness, changes in tone, or inco-ordination of the relevant muscles.

Dysexecutive syndrome A loose collection of cognitive and behavioural symptoms that include impulsivity, perseveration, disinhibition, and poor self-monitoring associated with damage to various locations in the frontal lobes.

Dysphagia Difficulty with swallowing, pain on swallowing.

Dysphasia Impairment of language comprehension or expression caused by damage to the relevant parts of the brain.

Egalitarian/ism The moral principle of treating all human beings as equals.

Emotionalism This is also sometimes referred to as 'emotional lability', 'inappropriate emotion' 'emotional incontinence', 'pathological crying or affect", 'pseudobulbar affect", and has been described in a wide range of neurological disorders. Its main clinical feature is an increased readiness to cry or, more rarely, laugh.

Empirical Based on observable evidence.

Epistemology The branch of philosophy concerned with how things can be known.

Executive function Those cognitive functions concerned with high level planning, organisation, and execution of goal directed behaviour.

Frontal lobe The portion of a cerebral hemisphere that is at the front.

Galen A Greek surgeon and physician living in the second century CE.

Gastrostomy A tube that is permanently inserted into the stomach so that nutrients can be directly introduced for patients who are unable to get sufficient nutrition by normal means. This can be done without the need for major surgery using percutaneous endoscopic placement (PEG).

Global aphasia Severe non fluent dysphasia with poor auditory comprehension and difficulty repeating what is said.

Goal attainment scaling (GAS) A method of combining and comparing progress on a number of varied goals by obtaining a standardised composite score based on a range of different measurement tools.

Hallucination A perception in the absence of an external stimulus.

Hemiparesis Muscular weakness affecting one side of the body (common after stroke).

Hemiplegia Paralysis of one side of the body (common in the early stages of stroke).

Herpes simplex encephalitis A viral infection of the brain.

Humanistic therapies A range of psychological approaches to counselling which aim to treat human beings as whole people in social relationship, with valid conscious intentions and goals, and who must take responsibility for their own wellbeing.

Hydrocephalus Accumulation of cerebrospinal fluid (CSF) in the skull ('water on the brain') that places the brain under pressure. It can occur as a complication of traumatic brain injury. Treatment involves draining fluid or managing the pressure on the brain using lumbar puncture or a shunt device.

Hypoxia Restricted oxygen supply. Where the brain is involved –'cerebral hypoxia' - restricted oxygen supply can lead to irreversible damage.

Idealism A very broad school of philosophy that asserts that we can only know what is in our minds minds –ideas - or that only minds or ideas exist.

Impairment A problem in body function or structure.

Interdisciplinary An approach to team working in which professionals of different disciplines cooperate and collaborate with each other towards common aims.

Intracerebral haemorrhage One cause of stroke –bleeding from a blood vessel inside the brain.

Kant, Immanuel (1724-1804). A German philosopher who brought together concepts that had previously been seen as in opposition in eighteenth century philosophy (reason and experience) in a new way, and was highly influential on the rise of new philsopohical movements in the nineteenth century.

Lateral geniculate bodies Two structures in the thalamus (just above the brainstem) which receive tracts of nerve cells carrying information from the eyes and relay the information via other tracts to the visual cortex.

Lesion A defined area of damage to the central nervous system.

Limbic system A collection of structures and tracts under the neocortex (and therefore phylogenetically more primitive) associated with the subjective experience and behavioural expression of affect and emotion.

Minimal (or low) awareness state An expression sometimes used to refer to patients who show many for the characteristics of persistent vegetative state, but at times seem to show some awareness of their surroundings. It is not a recognised diagnostic term.

Medial The side of a brain structure that is closest to the midline.

MRSA Methicillin resistant Staphylococcus aureus. A bacterium that is resistant to commonly used antibiotics.

Mill, John Stuart (1806-1873). A British economist and philosopher who was a strong advocate of the rights of the individual and of utilitarianism.

Morphology Physical form.

Motor cortex A strip of cerebral cortex towards the rear of the frontal lobe that is concerned with the generation of individual voluntary movements.

Multidisciplinary An approach to team working in which professionals of different disciplines work alongside each other towards a number of individual professional goals.

Multiple sclerosis A health condition affecting the myelin (fatty) sheath that insulates nerve cells thus allowing them to conduct nerve impulses efficiently. The course and severity of the condition varies, but it is generally associated with problems in movement, vision, and cognition.

Nasogastric tube A tube that is inserted through the nostril, pharynx and into the stomach in order to provide nutrition in patients who are unable to get sufficient nutrition by normal means.

Neglect (inattention) A loss of ability to pay attention to one side of space, usually the left, following brain injury that is not explained by problems with vision or hearing.

Neurological pain Chronic pain caused by damage to the pathways in the nervous system that are concerned with pain perception. It is a common consequence of spinal cord injury.

Neuron A cell of the nervous system. Outgrowths of the cell body –'axons' - connect neurons to other neurons. Bundles of axons in the peripheral nervous system are called 'nerves'. Bundles of axons within the central nervous system are called 'tracts'.

Neuropsychology The branch of psychology devoted to the connection between brain, cognition, and behaviour.

Non-maleficence The moral principle of not doing harm.

Nystagmus Small constant involuntary eye movements.

Occipital lobe The portion of a cerebral hemisphere that is at the back.

Optic nerve The nerve that runs from the back of the eye into the brain.

Orthopaedic Concerning the musculoskeletal system.

Orthosis/orthotic device A device that is used on the outside of the body (usually around a joint) to support a weakness or correct a deformity.

Parietal lobe The portion of a cerebral hemisphere that lies between the frontal and the occipital lobes (in the middle).

Parkinson's disease A chronic progressive health condition affecting the neurological system involved with movement. The main symptoms are tremor and rigidity. Cognition may also be impaired.

Participation restriction A problem in involvement in life situations.

Pathology A structural abnormality in an organ of the body (e.g. tumour, scar, area of dead tissue, shrinkage, or enlargement)

Peripheral nervous system (PNS) The cranial and spinal nerves.

Persistent vegetative state A condition arising from brain injury in which the patient shows no evidence of awareness of her interior world or the exterior world, and which persists for at least a month. It is associated with severe and widespread brain damage. It must be diagnosed by a team with specialist expertise in this condition. It may or may not be a permanent condition.

Petit mal A type of epileptic seizure in which there is a brief loss of awareness –'absence'.

Pharynx Opening of the oesophagus (gullet).

Phocomelia A condition that is present from birth characterised very short or absent long bones and fused fingers and toes.

Phylogeny/phylogenetic The evolutionary origin and relatedness of a species.

Pituitary gland A small structure at the base of the brain whose function is the secretion of hormones (e.g. growth hormone).

Post-traumatic epilepsy Epileptic seizures that occur following traumatic brain injury.

Post-traumatic amnesia (PTA) A period of disorientation and inability to recall events following traumatic brain injury. The duration of PTA gives a good indication of the severity of the injury.

Pre-motor cortex A strip of cerebral cortex towards the middle of the frontal lobe that is concerned with the combination of individual movements into more general large scale movements.

Procedural justice The principle of making and implementing decisions according to consistent and transparent rules.

Prosody The variation is stress, pitch, and rhythm of speech that conveys different shades of meaning.

Prosopagnosia The inability to identify familiar faces (that is to recognise family and friends on the basis of their facial appearance) following injury to the brain that cannot be accounted for by other visual disturbance.

Prosthesis/prosthetic device A structure that replaces a missing body part of cognitive function (e.g. artificial limb, memory pager).

Randomised controlled trial A research design in which the effects of a treatment are tested by randomly allocating participants to one or more experimental (e.g. drug) and control (e.g. placebo) groups.

Qualitative research methods Methods that rely on intensive study of small numbers of participants that focus on naturally occurring behaviour, often using semi-structured interviews or observations, and which deal with emergent themes and concepts.

Quantitative research methods Methods that rely on standardised methods of collecting numerical data, often with many data points generated by many research particpants.

Rationalism A philosophical approach which holds reason (deductive thought rather than experience) to be the only true basis of knowledge.

Receptors Specialised structures in the body or micro-structures within neurons that respond to stimulation (e.g. chemical, light, pressure).

Reduplicative paramnesia A rare delusion belief that a place has been duplicated in another location (e.g. that there are two identical versions of a hospital ward —one in the hospital and one in the patient's home.)

Retrograde amnesia The inability to remember events that occurred prior to a brain injury. This can often be patchy and with a temporal gradient, so that events closest to the occurrence of the injury are not recalled but events from earlier times recalled relatively better.

Rigidity (applied to muscles) The involuntary increase in resistance of a muscle when it is stretched (increased muscle tone).

Schizophrenia A severe mental health condition characterised by hallucinations, delusions, disorganised thinking, and affective disturbance.

Sensory cortex A strip of cerebral cortex at the front of the parietal lobe that is concerned with bodily sensations.

Serial plastering/casting/splinting Fixing of a joint that has been affected by contractures in positions of gradually increasing extension in order to increase range of movement.

Shipman, Harold (1946–2004) A British general practitioner who was convicted of the murder of fifteen of his patients in 2000, but is likely to have murdered at least 200 patients.

Spinal cord The part of the central nervous system outside the brain and inside the spine. It is concerned with the transmission of information necessary for bodily sensation and movement below the head and neck.

Stroke A general term referring to the sudden appearance of neurological symptoms following interruption of the blood supply to part(s) of the brain, either as the result of a blood clot or bleeding into the brain.

Supernumerary phantom limb A rare delusion that the person has an extra arm or leg. It occurs in conditions where sensation and movement in one arm or leg have been affected, for instance by a stroke.

Subarachnoid haemorrhage Bleeding into the subarachnoid space (in the outer layers between brain and skull), often a consequence of a malformation of blood vessels in the area.

Temporal lobe The portion of a cerebral hemisphere at the side. It lies in front of the occipital lobe and below the frontal and parietal lobes.

Thalamus A relatively large structure at the top of the brain stem nearest the cerebral hemispheres. It acts as a 'sensory gateway' to the cerebral hemispheres, receiving tracts of nerve cells from the eye, ear, and sensory receptors in the body.

Tinnitus A condition in which ringing, whistling, buzzing and humming are heard as if in the ears or inside the head.

Triage A system used in health care where resources are limited, often but not always in emergencies, to prioritise urgent cases.

Utilitarianism The principle that the moral value of an action is determined by the contribution of its consequences to the general good.

Vertigo A sensation of spinning when standing still.

Vigilance The ability to sustain attention for a long period of time on a detection task where the target does not occur frequently and is often unpredictable.

Visual cortex The area of the cerebral cortex in the occipital lobes that is concerned with the visual perception.

Visual field The area of space that can be seen when the eyes are kept fixed on one point.

Index